Generation Dances

A Caregiver's Journey

Mary Donovan Moeller

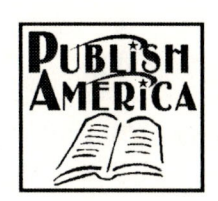

PublishAmerica
Baltimore

© 2006 by Mary Donovan Moeller.
All rights reserved. No part of this book may be reproduced, stored in a retrieval system or transmitted in any form or by any means without the prior written permission of the publishers, except by a reviewer who may quote brief passages in a review to be printed in a newspaper, magazine or journal.

First printing

ISBN: 1-4241-3874-4
PUBLISHED BY PUBLISHAMERICA, LLLP
www.publishamerica.com
Baltimore

Printed in the United States of America

I dedicate this book with love and gratitude
To my sister,
To Bill,
Our children and grandchildren,
To those woven into the history of our lives,
And to the memories of our ancestors.

Table of Contents

Foreword 7
Author's Note 9
Promise 11
Expanding Our Home 12
Checking History 19
Baggage Claim 24
Numbed Out 43
Get Married 53
New Life, Old Life 66
Onward 77
Answers to Prayers 91
All Together, Girls 108
An Indigo Bunting 114
One Cry 123
Welcome Folks 131
Hello Again, Will 137
A Final Toast 142
Lucking Out 152
Beyond Endurance 159
Speak Only to Grandma 168
Family Connections 172
Very Young and Very Old 178
Free Spirit 183
A Single Tear 187
Promise Kept 193

Foreword

As one who has shared most of the years, even if not most of the life of the author, I asked to welcome you to the discovery, the joys, the love this little book can offer. When I was young I built Sumerhouse "barehanded" in the mountains of Colorado and carved into the main beam "FOR MARY MY WONDERFUL WIFE." Many years have passed, and much has taken place since then. Only a little bit, a few little stories, from all those years is here. That may be enough to let you understand that what I once carved into a beam is now deeply carved throughout my being, changed only as language and time have evolved, so there it now reads "FRIEND."

I welcome you to glimpse what she has built from words and from herself, even as I would welcome those who cross the thresholds of the physical shelters built by my hands.

And may you have peace.

Bill

Author's Note

Certainly, I am not the only human on earth with a story. Everyone has a story they could tell honestly, from the perspective where their feet have touched our planet and from the perspective of cultural influence at a point in time.

I have chosen to tell my story as one example of how personal history can influence the care and attention given to dying family members. A possible caregiver would do well to appreciate the importance of the narrative, especially since more people may be tending such relatives in the future. Care giving can resurrect ancient feelings, as I learned nursing five dying seniors in our home. The elderly influenced our early years, and the baggage we carry often has bits of them in it. I fear much elder abuse flows from the weight of this baggage. The aged person and their junior caregiver could crash and knock at each other like bumper cars in an amusement park. Once we understand this, it is possible to benefit from the experience without dents and damage, and even to enjoy it.

As I wrote my personal account I could not avoid my training as a marriage and family therapist because this is a component of my present reality. I have tried to avoid diagnosing or psychobabble, which I dislike anyway, along with our family no-no of getting into another's head. When my youngest son read through an early version of this book he put a few "IHH" notations in the margins. This meant "in his or her head," something he knew I would not want. Within my family we have all labored to be honest about our thoughts, feelings, ideas, hopes, and dreams as we communicate, and recognize that we cannot know about each other through the projections of our fantasies but only through direct conversation.

I have not used last names or given identifying information, and even most first names have been changed. More important than the identity of anyone, including myself, is my hope that some may learn from this story and then become enriched through care of their own fading elders.

I want to thank the friends I have grown up with over the years, and with whom I am still growing up. My life without you would not be my life.

And I especially want to thank my husband and best editor, who opened to the process of my personal maturation. Learning to leave each other really free may be one of life's hardest lessons because we need each other so much, and we protect our fears so well.

Promise

Give me that hammer, child.
Come on, Bluegirl, hand it down.
No? You won't? You need me to tell the story first?
Okay, Okay, I'll tell it. But I will ask for it again. I will.

She is only an almost life-size painting of a sick child. Our *Bluegirl* has hung upon various walls in our home for well over four decades. Sometimes she frightens guests or grandchildren. She has witnessed our life and absorbed our feelings. She has heard our stories, our screams, and observed our tears. The raised hammer she holds above her head looks ready to launch destructively at the naked fetus-doll she dangles at her side from the other hand. Perhaps she is ready to destroy the forces that made her who she is. She wears a blue dress. Her eyes are wide and unforgiving. Yet like Pinocchio, she has earned reality and I'll try to help her. I will tell the story.

Expanding Our Home

The last musical notes from our daughter's joyous June wedding were still dancing through space when Bill and I began to build an in-law apartment onto our large brick house, and by September it became my mother's home.

My sister Ellen's family had given her years of devoted care, helping with shopping and doctor appointments. She never drove a car. Then her rent was raised exorbitantly, and she was less able to manage the stairs to her apartment. We thought the weakening of her legs was probably caused by arthritis.

Our mother was never capable of getting along with people, so settling her with other senior citizens would have been devastating for the elders in a community, and for my sister and me. We knew we'd have had to listen to a constant barrage of complaints! And certainly it was my turn to care for our mother. So Bill went to work, and her apartment was rapidly constructed.

Although Bill taught engineering as a professor in Lowell, Massachusetts, he had learned carpentry as a boy while helping his father. After losing a farm during the Depression, his industrious dad had changed occupations and had become a carpenter. Utilizing those childhood skills, Bill had built the original part of our home twenty years earlier.

Now, suddenly, we needed an attached but separate unit, providing an individual kitchen, bathroom, and distinct entrance with no direct access to the main house. Bill built in a cozy living room with a sliding glass door to a back garden. Only such a setup would preserve our own space. Caring for my mother without structured privacy would have been impossible. We provided her her own telephone line by which she could contact us anytime. There were phones in her kitchen and bedroom.

She moved into this establishment shortly after Labor Day, 1991, after our intense summer of preparation. Although Bill designed and framed the structure, the construction became a family project. Our youngest son, and new son-in-law, as well as many friends and relatives donated time and energy.

Initially my mother was an extremely stressful addition to our lives. She endeavored to create a world in her own image and likeness, and within that world she attempted to control all of us.

About a week after her arrival I went next door to find her collapsed on the floor.

"Get me a cigarette," she commanded.

"This doesn't look like a comfortable place to smoke," I replied.

"Goddamnsonofagoddamnbitch, do what I tell you," she screamed.

"I don't feel like doing anything for you when you talk to me like that," I answered quietly.

"Please," she said mockingly.

She got her cigarette and I went to get Bill, who was at home, fortunately.

She felt like a large jellyfish as we hoisted her into a chair, and then into my car for a trip to an emergency room. She had described feeling dizzy and nauseous, so I thought she might have some heart thing going on. It was not a heart problem but one of severe muscular weakness, which, along with her drooping eyes and facial mask warranted referral to a neurologist. He diagnosed *Myasthenia gravis*, a progressive, degenerative neuromuscular disorder.

The collar prescribed to support her head, and medication made it possible for her to hobble around the supermarket, which she enjoyed. I took her shopping one day each week, and out to lunch another. Since she loved to read and listen to music and the news; she was an interesting person. I would enjoy her one-liner sense of humor, which could give insight into others, though never into herself. As we talked, I tried to appreciate her. She'd always wanted my sister, her grandchildren, and I to appreciate music, poetry, and literature. But if we had missed something she thought we should know, she would call us nincompoops.

"Nincompoop, you nincompoop," she'd cry out and often follow her outburst by a crack over the head with the book containing the point of our ignorance.

As she settled into her new living quarters she played music endlessly, except when watching TV. She loved classical music and could operate tapes more easily than a CD device. Should she want me to hear a performance, so that I would be less of a nincompoop, she would blast it. The noise was inescapable, despite the house-wall separation. A common wall contained two windows from the original house that allowed me to check on her merely by opening one, but even when closed and curtained, they created an open channel for sound. Thus, during times when I was being musically educated, it was impossible for me to listen to anything else, or enjoy quiet, unless I went over and turned down the volume. My effort would not assure that her music would remain muted.

Had I not learned to separate my responsible care for my mother from how she responded to me, I would never have survived her living in an apartment attached to my house.

Just as it had been necessary to organize her physical environment, it was necessary to structure her mental world. She needed a clear sense of her limitations or she would simply push and push for more and more. She was insatiable. She was without any concept of the word "enough," so I would have spiraled down a black hole if I could not have balanced compassion with conservation of energy. And my psychological demise would not have been in her best interest, or mine, for that matter.

Although visitors often found her smart and funny, she was never any fun for Bill and me during her first year with us. It takes a relaxed space between persons for the eruption of laughter. Unfortunately, since she was always trying to control us within a world of her creation we constantly needed to remind her we had a world of our own. I was not bonded to her as a child to a mother, and her presence came with the baggage of miserable memories.

But life with my mother next door began to settle into a routine. Because I was still working as a family therapist, a court investigator, and teaching ethics for the evening school at the university, my schedule was tight. She would often try to change her shopping or luncheon time and rearrange my life, but she learned this didn't work.

Heading out to teach my class one night, I walked out my door and into the enclosed entryway as she hobbled out her door and stood leaning on her cane in the same entryway. Something was bugging her. It did not matter to her where I was going or how late I might become. I was commanded to listen while she began a loud, rambling diatribe. I told her that I didn't understand what she was talking about. She held onto the wall with one hand and with the other, lifted her cane to smack me.

"I don't care if you don't understand what I am saying. I understand what I'm saying," she screamed.

Bill heard her wordy attack and stepped into the common space. He said nothing at all but my mother immediately disappeared into her apartment and I continued on my way.

On a bright sunny morning soon thereafter, I'd tried to discuss some plans with her until she was began lashing vicious verbiage at me. Again she saw Bill coming towards us and lowered her voice to a reasonable tone. She never tried to bulldoze or antagonize Bill. This always amazed me. Perhaps she knew she'd met her match, even though there had never been any test or confrontation between them.

She no longer drank alcohol. She had not had a drink since she was allowed to leave an institution during the late sixties. This was certainly an admirable accomplishment given her old capacity to down a case of beer in an evening. However, she still smoked incessantly as she drank an endless pot of tea. My image of her remained unchanged; a formless lump endlessly slumped over a drink, dangling the smoke, while in her pajamas.

Then came the day I was forced to carry a candle into an unmapped corner of my soul. Although I often took her to Connecticut to visit Ellen's family, I was going alone this time. Any jaunt with her was an ordeal, and I did not have much time. I visited her kitchen to tell her I was leaving, told her who would be home to help her, and prepared to depart. She demanded she tag along with me, and I repeated that I was going alone for a short business trip.

She lunged after me. Holding onto the kitchen sink she lifted her cane into the air, her gaping orifice bellowing, "Yougoddamnsonofagoddamnbitch, I hope you rot in hell."

She started to swing her cane. As it descended towards my body I caught the tip. I realized that this person who had been physically abusive to Ellen and me was now much weaker than I. I realized I could push the cane with her on the other end of it back against a wall. Maybe I could push hard enough to kill the bitch and break her witch-head wide open.

Slowly and gently I put the tip of the cane on the floor.

"I will not be hit," I stated softly and left.

Slowly, I walked out her kitchen door, into the entryway, and through the door to my own kitchen. I sat down at my own kitchen table and put my head in my hands.

"Now you know you, too, are capable of becoming a persecutor. Now you know in your own heart that you are capable of killing another human being," I reflected to myself.

I shuddered at my desire for vengeance, and then relaxed knowing I had not hurt my mother but had simply acknowledged my feelings. Certainly we are more likely to act out destructive impulses when we can't allow ourselves to own them. But once admitted, we can choose to place them aside and focus on the positive. Sure wasn't easy, but I felt a renewed confidence in my capacity for discernment and commitment to remain gentle.

My mother phoned. She wanted to give me messages for persons in Connecticut. She was pleasant and said she'd see me when I returned. Violent behavior had not gotten her what she wanted, and she was smart enough to know it.

Such lessons are best learned before three years old. Both the neglected and spoiled child can wind up suffering from the same tendency to tyranny when not taught to respect the reality of others. Interesting how opposite extremes can produce similar results. When the small child learns to surrender unbridled narcissism in order to accept the loving limits of devoted guardians, the little one learns empathy and a sense of place within creation. These important lessons open the creativity of the child and enhance individuation. They free the child from the tyranny of self-obsession, and rescue any who would share life with this future adult from the trauma of tyranny. Of course, the child should be taught through relationship and never with any form of corporal degradation. Violence begets violence, and adult tyrants only create baby tyrants as they wallow together at the level of the two-year-old.

No one had taught my mother the important lessons of early childhood. I felt tremendous pity for her. Always aggressing for more and more, she was never able to be happy with what she had. She did not live in the present, but for what she could get out of another in the future. Therefore, she had no friends. The mutual zone between two friends is conceived by their respect and born from their liberty.

As months passed, her illness caused her legs to become weaker and her head to droop more. Cleaning her apartment was not easy for her. Because she had some phobia about germs, she wanted her residence scrubbed all the time. Although I had hired a cleaning service, she would still demand that I come right over and clean this or that. If I happened to be in the middle of some task when she called, I would explain what I was doing, and sincerely promise I would arrive as soon as I could. She'd swear at me because I was supposed to do what she said when she said it. I'd explain that screeching was not going to accomplish anything for her. She would swear at me again.

I would say, "I will not be sworn at," and then hang up.

She would call back and sweetly explain what she wanted done. I would repeat that I would arrive as soon as I could.

It seems I did this dance about one hundred times a week. Gradually she began to adapt and relinquish her attempts to dominate.

She seemed to enjoy her apartment and eventually, almost appeared happy. Watching various birds at the feeder and asking me to name the assorted flowers growing in the large garden outside her sliding glass door gave her much satisfaction. She read books about birds and flowers, and was proud of her knowledge.

It seemed she'd had to be structured like a small child so we'd be able to live together in peace. This had been exhausting, but our lives became more relaxed. Occasionally we were able to laugh together.

Checking History

The face of Doctor's only daughter wore the twist of a person about to unearth forbidden information. The power of her secret gave her power over me as I felt it coming. The woman had no genetic or emotional relevance to me until this moment. Her deceased mother had been Doctor's first wife, and my aunt his second, but she was about to make herself significant.

"You know," she said, "your father left your mother. They'd been together five years and he'd had enough of her. He'd known what a mistake he'd made on his honeymoon, but hung on. Finally, he left. Then he came back because *you* were coming."

I looked away from her snarled face. The event of my arrival in 1939 suddenly tasted like a bitter herb. I didn't focus on the empty bottle or her putrid breath. I felt blamed and invalidated.

About twelve-years-old, I had told my elders emphatically that I was no longer a child. After all, I could now bear one, so how could I still be one? According to myself, I was grown up, yet suddenly I wanted to find a grown-up I trusted.

I found Babe, my father's older sister. Was it true? Had he really left and returned because of me?

Babe could not lie. She became furious. "You were never supposed to know that," she bellowed. "How dare she take it upon herself? Who does she think she is?"

Babe's fury ranted on but did not change the fact.

I had just become responsible for everything. Still in the grips of childhood narcissism, I felt myself at the center of the universe. Therefore, I felt too much power and too much vulnerability. Everything was my fault. My father's thwarted freedom hung over me. Though I had always experienced his devotion and tenderness, always felt him to be my best friend; suddenly I decided I was his worst enemy. I had ensnared him and was responsible for his years of misery.

Yet my younger sister, my only sibling, and I were far more victimized. Children are always the most vulnerable under the power of a physically or emotionally violent person. My mother was a violent person.

The power of secrets has enthralled me since my pre-teen experience. Information can become a destructive force when transformed into a secret. A secret can be used to seduce a person into another's web, regardless of whether or not the information is accurate. The reputation of a person, family, or community can feel threatened if private matters become public, yet persons may not share the same cultural acceptance of what is a private or public matter. For my own life, I decided it was easier to live life openly and honestly. Better to be fallible and part of the imperfect human condition than try to hide. Others can smell dirty laundry even if it is concealed. But I would like to believe I could keep silent if another's life depended on my silence. Should I have lived during the Nazi reign of terror I hope I would have concealed Jewish children from them. There is real danger and there are real tyrants who commit real crimes against humanity, yet knowing the real from the imagined is often difficult.

As a therapist I keep secrets as part of my job. But I learned there are limits to such confidences when a client confesses a crime and then I am subpoenaed. This happened when a woman told me she missed visits with her children while transporting heroin by plane from one city to another in order to buy cheap and sell high.

And unfortunately, sometimes a secret lie creates its own reality. I like to believe that truth surfaces eventually, but even if it does this may not benefit the experience of an individual life or the lives of an unjustly rejected group.

A few years after my mother's death I discovered that a crucial piece of her identity had been a lie.

My mother was sixteen when she ran away from her miserable life in a Massachusetts convent boarding school to become a nurse at Misericordia Hospital in New York City. Her mother had died of leukemia when she was only four years old. She was then bestowed, for alternating stints, into the care of maiden aunts from both sides of her family. When I first met them, they were in their nineties and still complaining about having inherited the burden of this difficult child, whom they had eventually turned over to the often cruel discipline of nuns in a convent boarding school.

The sad story behind this, we all understood, was that upon the death of his wife her father had abandoned her; moved a few towns away; remarried, and produced six more children. She knew of him and his family but was excluded from their circle. She had been replaced. She believed this. It was a lie.

We tend to take the stories told to us about our families literally, as factual building blocks for our identities. Even when the stories are honest, it is hard for persons within families to accept that they experience each other and their histories differently. It can be difficult to become both unique and part of a community called family. Each becomes unique by embracing the value of her experience. It is relative and it is real. But what happens when a family discovers their mythology was built on a lie? A lie perverts the family, when people believe they can improve on factual reality with a fantasy. Some truth-creators may believe their motives are noble, or they may know they are not. It does not matter. Either way, truth has been crucified.

Truth began to appear one cold winter day when I drove into the

Boston area and buried myself in the Commonwealth of Massachusetts Archives for records before 1911 and the Commonwealth's other location for the Registry of Vital Statistics documenting marriage, divorce, birth, and death after 1911. I found my grandparents' birth, marriage, and death certificates and lots of amazing history. While doing this I felt cold and shaky, as if I was deliberately moving in on a ghost. I had a theory that my mother herself was the secret, but all checked out as acceptable to a traditional Irish Catholic family. All was recorded as she said it had been, until I came to her father, Joseph Lynch. He died in 1954 in Lowell, and was buried from a funeral home I had passed many times. His death certificate listed him as widowed from my grandmother, Nora Cronin. No mention of any other wife. The half-aunts or uncles my sister and I had planned to find didn't exist. At first I thought that a Mrs. Loretta Valliere, who was the informant of his death, might be some girlfriend with whom he'd produced all the missing relatives. I called O'Donnell's funeral home. They still had his record and sent it to me. Loretta was his sister; some aunt we never knew about. My grandfather had only one child, my mother, listed as Mary Lynch Donovan. My sister and I were his only grandchildren.

I will never drive past that funeral home without feeling cheated and angry, for my mother whose very identity problems hinged on the mythology about her father, and for my sister and me. We could have known a grandfather. My mother was told lies. Why? Certainly strange things happen during times of terrible grief, but there was never any reparation. The Cronins and the Lynches had about as much feeling for each other as the Sharks and the Jets in *West Side Story*! But to lie to the innocent child! Many have an identity built on illusions of grandeur and this is difficult enough for themselves and their children, but to build a child's identity on a lie is to damage rightful inheritance.

My grandparents, Nora Cronin Lynch and Joseph Lynch are buried together, side by side.

I went to their Massachusetts town and attempted to trace the story. I found the only living relative from either family, Loretta's daughter, now in her seventies. She knew her Uncle Joseph had never remarried or had another family. She laughed at the thought, because getting married and having any children at all was rare for both families. She had no idea why my mother would have been told such a tale. Maybe they were shamed by some family event. Perhaps there was a disagreement over money. I can only imagine, because the truth of what happened has been buried forever. Those who twisted reality are decidedly out of reach.

Thus, not surprisingly, my mother felt she was not wanted after her mother died. She remained emotionally arrested at about four-years-old for the rest of her life. She maintained the temper tantrums and the narcissism of a young child. However, she combined these with superior intelligence and brilliant manipulative talents she could use well when not pickled with alcohol or rage.

Baggage Claim

My father, Cornelius Rikardus Donovan, had left school following completion of the eighth grade to become a runner, a boy who transported message pouches for a Wall Street bank. There he met many businessmen who mentored him, which allowed him to work his way up through the ranks until he became a trust department president. Occasionally he enjoyed teaching business at New York University. This would be impossible in the twenty-first century, because a person would need a graduate degree and not an eighth-grade education.

With a medium build, an olive complexion, intense brown eyes and a very prominent nose, he looked as if he should have been wearing a yarmulke. Though a loyal Catholic, his Wall Street friends affectionately called him, "Duke, the Irish Jew." He was a quiet, relational, and very rational man with a philosophical sense of humor. And his life was devoted to maintaining a family for us, to the degree possible.

Like most fathers of our time with a developing professional life, he went off to work each morning, leaving the family with mother.

I'm told my first three years were peaceful because my mother could focus on a single child with the constant support of my father's two sisters, Babe and Nonie. Neither had children, and they loved playing with me.

When my sister arrived three years later, the added stress of a second child agitated my mother, and she became resentful of Babe and Nonie's close relationship to me and no longer wanted them around. Following Ellen's birth, we were usually alone with her. It was a world without humor. It was a world where I waited in terror for the next unpredictable blast.

I remember climbing some kind of changing table to look at my new sister. I peeked with horror at some black thing on her stomach. What was the rotten animal resting there? Suddenly my mother swung and sent me flying across the room. That was a very dangerous animal. I wondered if my sister was going to survive it.

Despite that thing on her belly she lived long enough to be baptized, and I enjoyed the family party. My daddy was home. Babe played the piano, and everyone sang. I giggled and played with Nonie, my dad's younger sister, who had taken over the care of Ellen and me for this day. I was so happy. I danced around and around and made our guests laugh. Baptism must be a good thing.

When my sister could sit by herself we played with a toy that stuck to the floor with a suction cup. It supported a heavy ball on top of a long coil that we could spring back and forth between us as we sat on opposite sides of the thing. One day, after I'd pulled the ball towards myself, it left my hand at the very moment Ellen leaned into the catapult. My sister hollered as my mother observed an expanding egg on her forehead. She smashed me and told me I'd killed my sister, before she threw me into a corner and disappeared to rush Ellen to the hospital. I crawled up to look out a window of our apartment about four stories above ground level. People walked rhythmically along the gray city street. Some were laughing together, others conversing, while still others meandered peacefully alone. They didn't seem to have any concerns. I wondered how I was going to live life as a murderess. Perhaps there was no hope for me.

Once again my sister survived.

A few months later, with Ellen in her carriage, the three of us went for a walk to some department store. Our mother went inside and left me outside to watch the lively eleven-month old. I held the handle of the big baby carriage very tightly with both hands, but I had a strong little sister. She climbed up and leaned over the edge. Soon she was on the ground screaming and growing another egg on her head. A patron ran in and found my mother, who suddenly appeared and then pounded me for killing my sister yet again. Customers came and went, stared at us, and said nothing. I was not yet four, but figured I'd deserved to be beaten. The passing world made no objection.

As an adult I have never been able to witness a child being beaten without intervening, often to my own detriment. The wisdom of this is questionable, because it is often a shamed parent who lashes out to blame a child. Should I cause a parent to feel more shame, the child could well be placed in more danger. I have wanted to let the little ones know someone out there believes they should be treated kindly. Perhaps there are ways to do this that can deflect the parental behavior with humor or help.

Soon after the street scene my mother was committed to a mental hospital for the first of many times. We visited her on weekends and benefitted from the loving care of Babe, Nonie, and our father. What a change! I was so happy. Life was full of laughter, games, music, and storybooks.

I never knew exactly why my mother went off to hospitals or why she returned. It was like a light switch being turned on and off. Throughout my youth she went away, and then she came back. When she left, Babe and Nonie would come; when she came back they would leave and no longer be present to us. They would go away out of respect for her space. Each time they disappeared my world became darker. The light switch had again been turned off.

At some point during my childhood, Babe came to care for us without Nonie. Nonie had married Arthur. That's what she called him, but Ellen and I were told to call him "Doctor." He was a surgeon who had been Chief of Staff at Miseracordia Hospital when my mother had arrived there to train for nursing. He had believed my mother was too young to handle operating-room stress and thought in-home nursing would be better for her. So he sent her to tend my father's dying mother. Doctor had already known my father's family, but this extended the relationship, and of course, his marriage to Nonie expanded it still further.

My mother was completely unpredictable. I would never know what would set off her physical attacks or round of verbal fury. Though she was never fun or funny, sometimes were more neutral than others. In defense, I developed an ability to memorize facial expressions and understand their meaning. This was a survival tool, and when my mother began to look like a witch, I got out of her way. She could not disguise her expressions, so my lessons in non-verbal language taught me nothing about those persons who smile to your face while also stabbing you in the back. For many decades should others present a pleasant mask, I believed the mask. Should people smile, I believed they liked me. The experience with my mother had trained me to observe unconcealed illness and potential violence, but not a theatrical stance. Only later did I begin to fathom the destructiveness incited by theatrically talented persons manipulating the emotions of others for their own ends.

By the time she returned from her first hospital stay, supposedly cured, we had moved from the New York City apartment where I'd danced for Ellen's baptism, to Bronxville, a suburb of New York City. Moving was to become a life pattern, because prior to my mother's release from a hospitalization, we'd change our address. Therefore, we moved many times, though I never understood the reason. Maybe my family was ashamed of her. Perhaps my father wanted to give her a fresh start. I never asked, and it was never discussed. Babe, Nonie, and our father talked as if nothing were wrong except that *The Mother*, as they called her, got "tired" and needed a "rest." Yet should I tell a friend about our circumstances I would be severely admonished by Babe and Nonie because they believed knowledge of family problems should remain at home. My family over-utilized a denial defense and pretended everything was "marvelous," thereby becoming isolated from community and support so desperately needed!

The white house in Bronxville, with its sprawling front lawn and little garden in the backyard, introduced us to a new environment. For city people this was rural America. I picked a big pot of thin string beans with my dad one summer and they will remain the best string beans I'll ever enjoy. A friend of my father's gave us a blue spruce as a housewarming gift, and it was exactly my height at the time. The tree became my friend, and sometimes I whispered into its branches what I could not say aloud. And within this house in Bronxville I was given a piano that became another friend. While touching its keys I could speak a language my relatives couldn't challenge.

When home after kindergarten, I'd play school songs by ear, which inspired my mother to take me for lessons. She desired I become a learned human being, for which I am grateful. I progressed rapidly, because I was recovering from two successive serious illnesses and couldn't do much else besides practice the piano.

During these afflictions I had overheard adults discussing my possible demise. First, doctors finally discovered my appendix had been rupturing a little now and a little then since birth. By the time they found the cause of my continuous low fever, I was in rough shape. Then, after that useless tissue was removed, they decided I needed my tonsils out in order to breathe correctly. Following the second surgery, a hospital nurse wheeled me to a sunroof where I promptly caught strep on my raw throat from another patient.

Doctor was in charge of the hospital and had removed my tonsils himself. He was furious and turned into the fire-breathing dragon I'd heard he could become when proper medical procedures were ignored.

His anger did not cure me. It was during World War II, and an antibiotic was not available. I fought off a fever near 107 degrees for days, and can remember shivering as I was immersed in freezing water. During this hospital stint in Manhattan, an air raid blared. The whole city froze in blackness. Alone in a room, I stared out a large window into nothingness. My world had become invisible as the mournful wails of the siren resounded. When the all clear rang out, a nurse rushed into my room.

"You poor little thing left all alone in the dark," she almost sobbed.

But I had not minded it much. Unlike my home, it was peaceful in this hospital, and I knew Doctor was nearby.

While recovering from these surgeries I was physically weak. I could not go to school, and should playmates visit my backyard, my mother would become hysterical and frighten them away. Apparently I was not to be exposed to anyone. The piano was a comfort to me, as I was not allowed to run outdoors.

It remained a comfort until I recovered. Then my piano teacher entered me into a children's Mozart competition in the city and I won first prize. Afterward my mother insisted I play the piano endlessly, with threats or thrashes if my enthusiasm seemed to flag for a moment. I felt so tired my fingers could barely move along the keys.

Suddenly, off she went to the hospital, and although I was happy that Babe returned, I had stopped talking. I had also stopped playing the piano. My father struggled to engage me in games and storybooks, while Babe told one joke after another. She played happy songs on the piano and sang and sang.

"In your Easter bonnet with all the frills upon it..."

I still hate that song.

Babe and my fathers' efforts brought enough happiness and warmth to my spirit that I began to speak again, but my focus was almost entirely on the meaninglessness of life. As I saw it, all any of us were ever going to do was die, so what was the use of bothering with anything? Babe found some *LIFE* magazine article depicting persons one hundred and two years gleefully sliding down banisters. I can picture her on the edge of my bed one night trying to cheer me up with the pictures of these seemingly eternal humans.

"Maybe they are one hundred and two, but they're still going to die," I answered solemnly.

It took much more warmth and happiness before I melted and could feel joy. Then the God so real to my father and to Babe became a Presence for me as for them. I felt Light, touching, warming and healing my spirit. They'd taught me we were created in the image of this Loving Presence and I attempted to see a love-image in each person, even my mother. I made my First Communion and felt this as a moment of unity to all the dancing molecules of our universe, because God was everywhere.

Fortunately for me, my childhood pediatrician had become more than just my doctor. She took me to concerts in the city and to FAO Swartz on Fifth Avenue. For years I kept a little Steiff chicken she'd bought me. When I was eight she sat me on her lap in her office and told me directly, simply and honestly that my mother was ill. She told me that my mother was never going to be capable of being a mother to me. I remember weeping and weeping from both sorrow and joy. Someone had finally told me the truth! My doctor, my friend, had been honest regarding reality my family could only deny. I knew it was the truth, and so I was relieved. My life at last felt real. From that day, I never expected anything from my mother. This lack of expectation was a great protection.

Subsequently, my child-theology projected God as a compassionate and healing doctor. Inspired by this devoted doctor, I wanted to become a doctor. She remained a support to me for many years, although my mother rejected her and wanted her dumped out of our lives as she had Babe and Nonie when I was younger. My mother always wound up in some kind of feud with everyone. The closer a person came to her emotionally or tried to understand her, the further she'd push them away. And it would be cause for wild smacking should I express appreciation for a person she'd rejected.

I realized my mother would soon return from the hospital because we moved. The piano came with us, but not my little fir tree. We had relocated to a three-story house in Queens without a front yard or room for a garden. Babe remained living with us, and took over the top floor. Ellen and I cheered because she wasn't leaving us this time. We felt less frightened and more hopeful.

We were all settled in the new house before our mother's Easter return. I had made a basket to welcome her, and selected many special little things to put into it. After a glance she pushed it aside. Then we went for a walk, she and I, and I'd hoped to enjoy her a little bit, but she began to scream at me.

I remarked, "I thought you were better now."

Big mistake! I was promptly hit on the top of my head again and again. People walked on by; once again no one seemed to care. For decades this was about as verbally brave as I ever ventured to be without apprehension.

As childhood plodded along, my dad was a generally a good father for me. He taught me to play chess, and many evenings we played the game by the hour. He took me to baseball games, and stemming from our old loyalty to the Brooklyn Dodgers, I still love baseball. We went out to dinner and talked. He loved music, and I touched the piano keys once again for him as he composed little things for me to play. We laughed. We talked about life. I attempted discussions about my mother with him. I told my dad I thought she was a self-centered child.

Once I was really upset and shouted at him, "She's selfish. She's totally selfish, and you won't see it."

"*The Mother*," he answered, "is basically good."

Forever and ever he tried to convince me she was a good person. Perhaps he'd envisioned some glimpse of that God-image he believed was imprinted within us all. Yet the voice tone with which he, Babe, and Nonie referred to *The Mother* whenever they discussed our family situation, managed to convey both a need for respect and a desire for distancing.

I grew as an independent child who wanted to stay far away from *The Mother* and her presumed basic goodness. Nonetheless, when with her, I listened to her endlessly. I wanted to see the face of Christ in her, and I also yearned to appease her so she would not treat me the way she treated my little sister.

My father was not a good father for my sister. Ellen would try to make *The Mother* into a good mother, for which she thanked Ellen by pounding her with any available item. You did not cross our mother.

She allowed no other perspective. She, alone, was ultimate reality. Throughout our childhood, our dad did not protect Ellen. But then, he could not even protect himself. When I'd watched *The Mother* lunge at him with a knife one evening while we still lived in Bronxville, he'd maneuvered us out of her way, but did not try to mellow her. He said nothing. He did not confront the experience of attack in any way. I assume my mother put the knife back in the drawer after she succeeded in getting us off her case. I don't know. If I'd asked I might have tickled the family denial defense. Did anything happen? *The Mother* was tired, and we must have upset her. Our fault.

As Babe tried to live her life from the third floor, our mother became more and more aggravated. She unscrewed and bounced light bulbs off the top of my father's head, calling him "Pope Cornelius," as he tried to teach me my catechism. She had become Protestant at this time, so the catechism was too Catholic for her. She wanted to protect me from *her Pope's* Church.

And yet this may have been my mother's unrecognized, unappreciated drive for her health. I believe we are always striving for greater health, although the ways we go about it often cause us more problems. Our family and friends may feel challenged by our actions or new beliefs, and often misunderstand behaviors that reflect personal growth. Although my dad was not a rigid, dogmatic, or morbid Catholic, was even Jewish philosophically, he was still an Irish Catholic who believed he had married another one. For my mother to have become Protestant and reject Holy Mother Church and even invite the Protestant minister to our home was diagnosed as a symptom of her instability. In our society today we can witness a myriad of examples of confused or challenged persons diagnosing others into some comfortable condition that makes sense out of them, or attempts to control them into some box. One friend seemingly mistreats another and suddenly the friend has "borderline personality disorder." I become irate at all the non-professional diagnosing and am sure the root of this anger is my family's constant diagnosis of my mother. As long as the focus could be her mental health, though certainly deficient, the deficient mental health of the rest of the family could be ignored.

But my mother's experience of Catholicism had little in common with my father's. Her maiden aunts were cold and extremely superstitious people. One of them, a Mary Cronin, came to care for Ellen and me twice when we were little, while Babe was traveling or ill. We created a game called *Mrs. Bitta*, reflecting our dealing with this cold, severe and controlling woman who would throw our clothes out the window if we had not picked them up precisely when she had told us to pick them up. Then she ordered us outdoors to get them. Once we refused and told her to get them herself. I preferred *The Mother* to *Mrs. Bitta*. Unlike my father's Irish immigrant family, my mother's Irish family had lived in the States for generations and worked in the textile mills. Somehow Irish Jansenism may have combined with New England Puritanism to create an especially deadly duo.

During the endless childhood hours when I had listened to my mother's monologues I heard her mention the convent boarding school where she had been placed when these aunts decided she was a difficult child. Then the year before her death she had wanted to visit the place, and I drove her to where it had been because it was less than one hour from the house. The massive red brick structure on a hill, no longer a convent boarding school, stared down at my car in the parking lot. My mother sat and stared back. Then she lit a cigarette in my car, prohibited because I am allergic to smoke. I didn't say anything.

Suddenly I wondered what had happed to her in there. I knew she had spoken of being made to kneel for hours on cold tile with no padding for her knees, as one punishment for transgressions. There were others.

I wrote to the order of nuns. She did attend that boarding school, and I obtained a few of her grades. She never graduated and disappeared at sixteen when she took off for New York City.

Whatever my mother's stand against Catholicism might have resolved for her, she was not free to discover. *Her Pope* barred the Protestant minister from returning to our home.

Yanked back into the box of religious correctness without language for definition or a confident sense of self, *The Mother* threw dishes and pots. She lashed out at my sister when I was the only other person at home to witness her violence. As a child myself, there was nothing I could do. I was powerless to control my mother and protect Ellen, and I felt guilty for being so powerless. It's not that I would have been safe from her fists, but mine was a flight and not a fight defense. I took off into music, books, and literally out the door! Ellen was angry with me for being so powerless and seemingly obnoxious with my silent disappearing acts. She told me I was not the kind of older sister she wanted and occasionally kicked or tickled me to death to prove it. But we were both powerless kids trying to survive through our own styles.

Our mother drank. My sister came to notice this and poured the stuff down the drain. She worked hard trying to reform *The Mother* into a good mother. No pediatrician had ever told her it was hopeless. Because she was a fighter and not one to run away, she was blamed more than I for upsetting *The Mother*, so fixing her probably seemed in her best interest. Ellen was whacked with the empty bottle or anything else for her efforts.

A temper tantrum was in charge of the home. I was out of there as much as possible.

The Mother was in command until a fateful evening when she apparently became fed up with Babe residing on the third floor. Babe was a high school English teacher and would grade her students' papers while Ellen and I read or finished homework on her floor. We liked it up there. It did not feel like our home but Babe's. Perhaps our mother was jealous, but whatever her motive she came upstairs after Babe. Our safe haven was invaded. Babe went out to greet her pleasantly at the top of the spiral staircase. Then Ellen and I watched in horror as our mother attacked and tried to flip Babe over the railing, almost hurling her into the abyss that terminated on the ground floor. A moment before success our father appeared and stopped her.

Again, *The Mother* was off to the hospital. This time I figured I knew why.

Frightened and shaken, I lay, trying to sleep, in my darkened bedroom. Then the apparition of a large, multicolored picture of the Holy Family appeared on the wall in front of me, just below the ceiling. Mary, Joseph and Baby Jesus interacted with excruciating tenderness. The joy and tenderness that flowed among them increased the light around them. Then I saw figures at the edge of the light that looked like ugly gargoyles. They loomed in various shades of gray and moved with jerky hostility. Their faces sneered many hateful expressions as they snapped at the Loving Ones. The little family did not notice the monsters, and the monsters could not travel into the light. They were stuck snarling in the shadows.

Years later when I learned that Helen Keller had said, "Keep your face to the sunshine and you cannot see the shadow," I remembered it and felt I knew what she had meant.

I can still see the bedroom, that wall, and the images today in the twenty-first century. Certainly I understand the power of my stress and feelings of loneliness as we helplessly watched Babe's danger. Yet I experienced a love and acceptance never encountered in my life. I had been taught principals of compassion through our family's religious tradition and believe that I could have had a similar experience of compassion through other images if I had been raised in a different culture. There may be many paths to this same awareness. Mine was a big boost for a troubled child.

We moved, of course, before my mother was released from the hospitalization following her assault on Babe. Another house gone, more friends abandoned, as we settled into an apartment near the East River on 23rd Street in Manhattan. Babe was no longer with us.

When our mother did come home, my sister and I were sent to a Holy Child boarding school in New Jersey, where I spent the seventh and eighth grades. There I experienced tender nurturing from inspiring priests and nuns. I would have had a very different life if I had bumped into some of the abusive clergy who have been so damaging to so many. *The Mother* remained my sole attacker, and by confirming her limitations, my pediatrician had helped soften her effect. No one overpowered the sanctity of my inner space, or exposed my vulnerable child-self to adult eroticism. If I'd had to toss more chaos into my emotional stew, I don't imagine myself surviving.

The clergy I was privileged to know attempted to live lives of loving service. They reinforced my father's lessons about finding God everywhere, and seeing the face of Christ in everyone. I desired to become a nun. Living with those attempting to love God directly had been an amazingly peaceful experience. The light bulbs stayed in their sockets, people did not raise their voices, and knives were used to prepare food. Becoming a medical missionary could combine this vocation with medicine, so I set a new goal.

Safe with these devoted religious I was able to ask a trusted nun if I were an awful sinner to wish my mother dead. Sin was a dogmatically and legalistically defined entity capable of removing a soul from the love of God. There were the deadly mortal ones, and those venial sins that still needed to be owned and confessed. For Irish Catholics what constituted a sin, and then defining the category of the sin were topics for many discussions. Certainly before weekly confessions a personal decision was needed regarding guilt. The negativism of sins, *withouts*, from the Latin root of the word, was emphasized more than the positive message of Christ to love God, neighbor and self. And unfortunately we were not taught that we're all supposed to be full of *withouts* because we are humans and not gods. Yet I was comforted by the nun's response. She said I was only asking compassionate release for my tortured mother. But I feared my motives were not entirely noble, so worked on my capacity for compassion.

My peaceful years were Ellen's nightmare. As a fourth grader, she had entered the Holy Child boarding school with me. Almost immediately, she developed severe nosebleeds. Our mother wanted Ellen returned to New York City. She said Ellen was not safe in the country and needed to be near big hospitals. Ellen fought and begged our father. She pleaded not to be left alone with her mother. I fought and begged my father. I told him there was a fine hospital near the school. He said *The Mother* was a nurse and knew best. He would not cross her!

Maybe our father had never seen enough of her violence towards us to really understand how much Ellen and I needed protection. I remember our mother behaving more kindly towards us when he was home. Children may absorb their family dynamics more realistically because parents do not defend against revealing themselves before their children as they defend against doing so to each other. Ellen and I were not clobbered in front of our father, though he was threatened in front of us.

Our mother could restrain her ranting when the telephone rang. Though she'd been shrieking at both Ellen and me, as she lifted the receiver her tone would reform completely into a high, sweet chime. This would give me the feeling that there were persons in the world deserving of some kindness from her, but my sister and I were not among those blessed. If she was speaking to our father, I'm sure he thought, and wanted to believe, everything was going well.

So often we believe what we want to believe and don't even collect the evidence we almost trip over that would elucidate our fallacies. One bad day I photographed *The Mother*. These pictures reflected quite accurately the face confronting Ellen and me continuously. She was so into her raging that she didn't seem to notice I had snapped the pictures. One day I mustered enough courage to show them to my father. I wanted to give him some feeling for our experiences when he was not around. He took them out of my hand and ripped them up. He said nothing. I was dismissed and felt blamed, as if I'd created rather than recorded our reality.

Ellen told me that the worst day of her life was the day she awoke and found me gone. I had been sent back to boarding school while she was to remain in New York City. She attended seven schools during the next few years when she was home alone with the intoxicated temper tantrum. She said that during this time our father did not come home early. Often he may not have come home at all. Ellen became so traumatized that she could no longer hear, as once I had not been able to speak. She was given hearing aides.

Bookstores today offer many books on the causes and effects of PTSD (Post Traumatic Stress Disorder). The numbing effect, the startle reflex, I know them all. Recently I was hiking down a mountain trail when another hiker suddenly and quietly arrived near my right shoulder. As I startled, my right arm flew up and unintentionally punched her in the nose. I apologized, as did she for believing she'd frightened me. I am still automatically on guard against *The Mother*. Although many have this type of reaction in common, every traumatized person will aim for inner balance through avenues that work for him or her, such that my sister and I closed off different channels.

I felt continuously sad about Ellen and powerless to help her. My father had not listened. Perhaps to some degree we all protect our illusions at the expense of others or blind ourselves to the obvious because it is too painful. Some type of survival may depend on this, though it often threatens our long-term survival or the welfare of others. I could not imagine what our father was thinking or feeling. A mother who had threatened his life and nearly killed his sister was not fit to have a child alone in her care. Yes, he was my sensitive, tender daddy. I loved him. I adored him. Yet he could not, would not, listen.

When I became an adult, Babe and Nonie confided that my father had wanted to gain custody of Ellen and me. They said he was forever asking his lawyer friends how he could do this, but they advised him that a mother was almost always given custody of the children no matter what was wrong with her. Nurturing was considered to be a natural instinct given to women and lacking in men. Apparently he was afraid to go to court for fear of losing.

It is an easy mistake to evaluate past generations in the light of present-day research and awareness. During my childhood there were few legal protections for the safety of children. The mentality that allowed my elders to believe they could keep family violence secured within our walls also reflected the belief that parents controlled the treatment of children within the family. Children were chattel, family property. An outsider would not interfere with the treatment of another's child any more than they'd move another's car. This is why I could be cracked on a city sidewalk without anyone interfering. There were laws to protect animals before there were laws to protect children, so I may have been better off as a dog, though the one dog we owned for a short time did not make out too well.

I do not accept corporal punishment as a means of parental discipline. Nonetheless there is a difference between spanking and child abuse. Children need to learn limits and discipline, and I firmly support non-violent ways of teaching these. Yet children recognize the difference between a spanking for a particular transgression that is followed by discussion and fierce, unexpected blows that are outlets for adult anger and frustration. Such explosions blame and shame the child for adult inadequacies. They do not teach personal responsibility and limits but limit the child's sense of value for him or herself.

Finally Ellen was sent back to the Holy Child boarding school in time for seventh grade. Still unable to hear, the highest mark she could attain was a forty. Slowly, this child who would eventually become an excellent nurse, began to heal. She remained at this school through High School.

When Ellen returned to the Holy Child Sisters I was brought back to 23rd Street. From the apartment, I walked to school, an academically excellent Quaker high school located near Gramercy Park. Most of the teachers and students were Jews, with whom I discussed cultural differences within a school philosophy of peace and acceptance. Science and math were favorite subjects and good preparation for my medical missionary objective. Though the school was nearby I never wanted to invite friends home, so I didn't accept invitations to visit them. Usually I returned after school to drop off books and check things out. If my mother screamed or was inebriated I would leave and explore the streets. Since she was almost always agitated or intoxicated, though never both at the same time, I rarely stayed home.

I met all kinds of people on the streets of New York City, friendly, smiling folks, and secretive, strange ones.

When I rode a subway uptown from our neighborhood to sections with more cultural opportunities, the subways were dark, dirty places with crevices carved here and there. Often, as I turned a corner towards a train, some weird man who had noticed my solo travels would step out of a shadowy place saluting me with his male anatomy. I believe I confronted these waving appendages in every color, size, and shape.

The aspiring missionary that I was would attempt to look the guy in the eye. I would raise my right hand and bless him, in Latin, of course. Making the sign of the cross towards him I would say, "*In Nomine Patris, et Filii et Spiritus Sancti, Amen.*"

Generally, he would turn away from me.

The Missionary was convinced these souls simply did not understand Love. Only years later did I realized how lucky I was not to have been shot in one manner or another!

As for the creeps who pressed themselves into me on a crowded bus or subway car, they did not get blessed. They had not left enough space. They were just dismissed with a loud, "Excuse me," as I pushed on through knotted flesh to another place.

Despite negative experiences these were the years I came to love New York City as my home, caretaker, and educator. I was immersed within a wondrous diversity of human culture as I explored many ethnic areas. I visited museum after museum, and relished operas and plays, which anyone could attend for a fifty-cent standing-room ticket. Because I loved music and enjoyed singing, I imagined myself in one operatic role after another as a way to learn something of my emotional self.

At home out of the home, I sometimes visited a priest friend and walked the streets of his poverty-stricken parish with him. I had met him at the Holy Child boarding school when he arrived to visit his sister. A Jesuit on leave from his station as a chaplain during the Korean War, he organized a slide show of his ministry there, and a few of us were invited. In the midst of war he had taken a picture of a single blue flower. I was amazed that he could find beauty in the midst of such horror. There were slides of the orphanages he had founded for fragile-looking children. He loved these pictures, as he did those of the beautiful girls he had pulled out of prostitution to work the orphanages. Nothing human shocked him. He was my example of living compassion.

Realizing how extremely important Father Frank became to my personal equilibrium, I can only shudder at the present-day awareness of extensive, concealed sexual abuse by priests. Children were sacrificed for the protection of the powerful. Although there is nothing new about that, it is all the more horrifying when such exploitation hides itself behind holiness and is meted out by a person called, "Father." This deceit adds an incestuous twist to an already pathetic crime. Those not able to practice the celibacy they took on could at least pick on people their own age. But herein lies a problem because, although these are physically mature adults, they may be emotionally thwarted children.

Father Frank, luckily for me, was able to bestow great physical tenderness without crossing that hard-to-define line that would communicate the gimmie-gimmies. Children who have suffered violation may not be able to feel that line. I was never sexually violated, and my experience of holistic tenderness left me free as an adult to evolve my sexuality without inner feelings of degradation. Although communication of a healthy sexual dynamic was non-existent in the asexual worlds of my home and school, I was not deprived of tenderness. I am concerned that the modern awareness of the damage done by sexual abuse may have created a sterile environment, which could block children from the experience of tender teachers, priests, doctors, and even parents. The loss of relaxed hugs may become as damaging as the horror of sexual abuse.

Following my excursions on the city's streets, I would usually get back to the apartment before my father. Apparently he was at home out of the home also. We were both avoiders, not fighters like Ellen. Occasionally he would drink too much and think he was some Rabbi. He was a harmless, philosophical Rabbi, but no use to me. We couldn't even play chess.

This Rabbi returned one evening with a bunch of tipsy friends. Eventually I decided they should go home. I placed a few drinks on some kind of trick tray rigged with three chains and a handle so it could be whirled in loops without spilling the drinks. I walked into the living room and offered them each another scotch as I twirled the tray. The men looked dazed and decided it was time to leave.

"You're very human," my dad said later.

Throughout my life his simple statement has remained my most treasured compliment, whether it was supposed to be a compliment or not.

My academically excellent Quaker school required homework. I would arise at four in the morning when the house was quiet in order to accomplish the task. My grades did not reflect problems. After a geometry class I would explain the subject to a bunch of boys who simply could not understand it through the accent of our foreign-born teacher. To this day I remember the history teacher's comment during the World Series that there would be hope for our troubled world as long as everyone could stop everything and enjoy a ball game. I remembered my trips to the ballpark with my dad and felt hope. I was president of my sophomore class and enjoyed having friends within a co-ed environment, even though I didn't hang out with them after school. But eventually my father caught me studying before dawn and decided I was under too much stress. He sent me back to Holy Child for the last two years of high school.

Ellen and I were together again for the first time in years.

I spent two peaceful years with my natural sister and the Holy Child sisters. I took pleasure in my studies and looked forward to joining religious life. The school offered excellent piano and voice instructors who coached me for solo performances in both disciplines. Once again music became a deep personal satisfaction. Sometimes I took a train to the city for a long weekend but was always happy to return. With relative ease I graduated from high school and was accepted at the College of New Rochelle. It was time for change.

Numbed Out

    I packed for college remembering my graduation ceremony from Holy Child. It had shimmered with girls in white dresses singing beautiful songs to Our Lady, proclaiming our innocence to the world. We were holy children.
    Once settled into New Rochelle, I persisted with my childhood plan to become a medical missionary and enrolled in the appropriate courses. But the heavens play games with human plans. My father became ill during this freshman year. At first we thought he had a bad virus, then polyps on his larynx but eventually he was diagnosed with cancer of the throat.
    I declared my major as English. This required no lab work and enabled me to place books into a bag, make the rounds of the different hospitals, and at least complete a college degree. I had three hospitals to visit. Along with my father's, Doctor was debilitated with Parkinson's disease, and my mother was back in her mental hospital after yet another terrifying experience.
    I had ridden the commuter train back to the city from New Rochelle to check on how she was doing, home alone in the

Manhattan apartment. I turned the key and walked into a nightmare. She was not dressed. Beer cans were everywhere. Burned cigarettes were piled high. She was drunk and disheveled. Food was left here and there. Slumped over a telephone, she believed she was talking to someone. She barely noticed me. She would not answer me. My father was no help. I didn't know what to do. I called Doctor's son-in-law, who worked nearby.

When this short, obese, paternalistic man walked through the door, my mother more than noticed him. She grabbed the largest knife from the kitchen drawer, and went after him. Although he had the huge advantage of weight, she seemed to have taken on the strength of six men. I watched as they struggled on and on for what seemed like hours. Often the knife almost gored his neck. I wondered what would happen if he lost. Perhaps I would be next. I thought about doing my usual disappearing act, but the door out of the apartment was on the other side of the fight. Eventually he overcame her, and took the weapon away.

He filed a report. To my knowledge a police report had never been filed on her before. Medical attendants wrapped her into a white straightjacket. I rode with her in an ambulance to Bellevue Hospital, where they put her, naked, into some bathtub. Her moans and wails ground into my soul. She looked pathetic, like some combination of a whipped animal and a lost little child, as she would look about two years later when they escorted her to my father's funeral.

After leaving my mother groaning in the tub at Bellevue, I caught another train back to New Rochelle. I returned to college life. I'm sure I did not look as if I'd had a bad weekend, but an invisible scar had frozen my spirit for years to come.

Following my mother's departure, Babe moved into our apartment and cared for her brother between his hospital stays.

During one of my dad's early hospital admissions a group of Holy Child nuns arrived to visit him. They pinned various medals and religious relics onto his clothing and bedside because they really wanted a miracle that would put their religious founder in the running to be declared a saint. I can still picture my father's patient, amused face as he acquiesced to their demands. He never asked for miracles, though I'm sure he believed God could pull one off. My dad was happy to consider himself part of the natural world and taught me that how I played the cards life dealt was what mattered. He believed we are a part of God's creation as any other species is, though we had been blessed with the consciousness to appreciate our place and our creator. This appreciation bestowed a responsibility to respect all that was used for food and shelter.

Through his philosophical outlook I learned that neither money nor prestige made a person superior, because we were one interdependent family of human mortals. I'm sure his attitude inspired his treatment of others, which was as kind to a janitor or waitress as to some important client. He knew we could die at any moment should we sicken with terminal illness, be hit by the wrong truck, or bump into a dangerous animal. That's just the way it is. Through accepting this fragility we could learn our place within creation. Powerless, we could rejoice in a tender embrace, a child's smile, a helping hand, or an honest tear. We could learn gratitude for the strength of human love, for fresh clean water, for shelter from a storm and a warm bowl of soup.

At times I wondered if God really was such a great lover when nasty tricks were inflicted on the innocent. In the face of our family violence I had blamed *The Mother*. Who could be blamed for a deadly cancer that was whittling my precious father to nothing, although these days medical science recognizes the deadly duo of his expensive, smoky scotch and cigars! The nuns had asked God to come on down and fix the problem, give them their miracle. So if God didn't, He'd turned His back. It was God's fault. Not very loving.

Babe used to shake her fist at God. She had no fear that her honest anger would turn to rage or violence, something more likely to happen when anger is not correctly accepted. Her open anger was her gift to God, a kind of prayer. Did God answer her as He answered Job?

"Where were you when I founded the earth? Tell me, if you have understanding…"

(Job 38:4)

With Job we scream out in anger at our suffering. We desire to be above creation, not but a part of a natural world; although even when saved from disaster we recognize we are no better than those who were not saved. Our insignificance insults us. And our drive for greater power than is our due leads to the devastations we inflict upon each other in so many bloody and bloodless ways.

My father no longer had a voice through which to express anger or anything else. A hole in his neck, through which he breathed, needed frequent suctioning. About eighteen months after his diagnosis the doctors found cancer in his lung. He wrote on his tablet and lifted his comment for me to read.
"Well, can't live without air. Need air to breathe."
Though dying, he disappeared while I was home for a weekend. Where was he? Babe and I were frantic. How did he manage to take off?
Eventually he returned, writing tablet in hand, with the few bucks he'd won at the Belmont Racetrack. Horses were in his blood, perhaps because his ancestors had raised racehorses in Ireland. He would never bet more than twelve dollars and would never take me with him. I seemed to serve as a surrogate son when it came to chess, baseball games, and lessons about Wall Street bargaining, but became his lady when it came to the racetrack because I was never allowed to go.
When my dad was very near death, a young colleague he'd mentored came to our home to say good-bye. As my father sat wrapped in blankets, propped in a comfortable chair, the man knelt before him and put his head on my dad's knee. He wept like a baby, and then left our home for the airport. A few hours later we learned he'd been killed in a commercial airline crash. I sat in silence. With his tears still wet on my father's blanket, the fragility of human life overwhelmed me. Suddenly, I desired to live my life ready to leave this world on a moment's notice. Aware of how quickly a loved one could be taken from me, teasing out interpersonal harmony became a lifelong need.

Following the 9/11 attacks on the World Trade Center there were many stories of ultimate farewells by persons who had thought they were sending loved ones off to work as usual. Many were grateful for a special hug, an extra kiss. I felt sadness for those relationships poisoned forever with hostility. I knew those stories were not being told, but existed. They always do. And the consequences of antagonism will burden the living for their remaining days and may even burden the dead for all we know. Best to resolve our petty conflicts and part peacefully from our brothers and sisters at all times.

My father was to die at the end of my junior year.

While attending a class I suddenly felt I should return to the city. My father was comatose when I arrived at his hospital bedside.

I talked to him and called, "Daddy."

He opened his eyes and looked at me. His hazed, brown eyes seemed to say, "Thanks."

He'd always wanted me to call him "Daddy," but I'd insisted on "Dad." The "Dad" kept a bit more distance between us that felt comfortable. He had no wife, that's for sure, and I think I filled some need for psychological closeness. There was never a seductive nuance in our relationship, though a tension evolved as I reached sexual maturity. This tension could have been a relaxed and natural part of life between a father and daughter under normal conditions, but our conditions were not normal. I became used to living in tension with my unmarried father and caught his tightness like the flu. I maintained physical distance in the midst of psychological closeness, and my formal language fit the lifestyle.

If he'd been a hugging sort he could have kept distance and remained relaxed. I did not learn the value of hugging from my physically aloof Irish family. Both Father Frank and his sister were physically affectionate, though Irish, a lesson that warns against stereotyping, but the Irish, as I generally experienced the culture, understood the relaxing capacity of whiskey more than that of touch.

My tension eased in the face of death, as I said, "Daddy."

I softened with the surrender of formality and my father's sign of gratitude.

He died that evening.

After his death I lost the devoted protection he'd been able to provide. Feeling abandoned, I reacted to my life's traumatic stress. The shock of witnessing the knife attack after years of exposure to unpredictable family violence had taken its toll. The inability to feel love or any other strong emotion was a component of this disorder for me, and complicated and prolonged my grief reaction. I could transmit emotion through my dependable piano, and expressed anger through music but otherwise did not recognize feeling. During high school I had played a Mozart sonata in concert, learned List's *Liebestraum*, and Debussy's *Clair de Lune*. Now I banged out Beethoven's *Pathetique*. It was Beethoven's anger, not mine. I was emotionally anesthetized.

Despite his weaknesses, my dad had been my closest friend. With his death I lost the support to go into medicine. I was alone, with a little sister boarding at Holy Child. I was alone except for Babe and Nonie.

Babe, my father's soft and chubby older sister who had always moved into our home to care for us whenever our mother was moved out, was our childhood salvation. I recall walking home from fourth grade to find an ambulance outside the door. I remember feeling happy because I knew Babe would be back. We were always so relieved to see her. She loved us, cooked for us, helped us with homework. She mended our clothes and would rub our heads. We sat around the kitchen table with her and talked and talked. More than anything, we laughed. She found humor in anything and everything. Babe never married, devoting her life to service for us, as previously for her parents.

With our mother institutionalized for attempted murder, and our father deceased, Ellen and I now became Babe's children. We changed our address to a less-expensive apartment a few blocks away on 20th Street. This apartment was still near the East River, and we could even see it from our windows. The three of us were a family.

Her new role was very hard for Babe now that there was "no man in the house." Throughout our childhoods, my father had always been there whenever she had arrived. She was also tired from caring for my dad during his last days, and was grieving the loss of her only brother.

Babe felt she had to protect Ellen and me, and I was a difficult one to protect. Though traumatized, I functioned well enough intellectually, and had years of experience living independently on the streets of Manhattan.

I accepted a summer job in 1960, the very summer following my father's death, taking the Census for the US Government, and because I did so well, was given a second assignment. After all, I knew those city streets! Trained to go everywhere, I was the only female included in a group to search for lost people at all hours.

One evening, after pursuing missing persons in a known house of prostitution, I bumped into Babe as I headed for the subway station. Poor, frightened Babe had been attempting to follow me around to assure my safety. I really didn't want to lose her to heart failure, so I pledged to work during daylight hours. I had a small enough family. This agreement pleased Nonie. She believed Babe should have curtailed my travels long before.

Nonie was thin, bony, angular, and an energetic second grade teacher. She was rather bossy, but her smile could glow a celestial sweetness. Her husband's Parkinson's was worsening, so she had little energy for Ellen and me. However, Babe always called her to discuss any decision.

The phone conferences between my father's older and younger sisters became the forum that promoted my becoming a teacher. Teaching was a good profession for a woman until she married and had a family. Medicine was for men.

Doctor, of course, was male. All his medical colleagues were males. Nonie and the other wives of physicians remained separate. They reveled in some esteem granted them for having married a doctor. Their place was to support these mighty ones, and to fulfill their human potential through the successes of their husbands, or so it seemed. The doctor was close to God, as was the priest, and maleness made this more possible, somehow.

The pediatrician, Olive Bosworth, whose honesty with me I have already credited with my childhood sanity, was a woman. Gentle and kind, she was not a mighty one but had nurtured and taught me while touching both body and soul.

And during the teen years another pediatrician, a brilliant, forthright woman named Hedwig Koenig, came to our New York City apartment many a time to rescue Ellen and me. Today, she would have had to report these rescues. At that time there would not have been anyone to accept a report. Her assistance was powerful and to the point, not apologetic and subservient, yet she displayed no interest in her own power other than her capacity to soothe and heal.

I can picture the brochures I'd collected and saved picturing women doctors in the missions comforting the sick. These medical nuns did not look like mighty ones.

Actually, Doctor seemed to care less about his being a mighty one than did Nonie. A slight, shy, somewhat stooped man, he had developed a new thyroid surgery that left only a thin scar on the neck. It was safer and a cosmetic improvement over previous procedures. He was devoted to his patients, though he maintained a professional aloofness towards them all.

Many of his patients paid him with presents. Babe, Ellen and I joined Nonie and Doctor for elaborate Chinese dinners delivered to their home. When we'd gather for Thanksgiving, he'd carve a huge turkey with his operating room knives without a hint of obvious humor, as we sat together beneath the magnificent crystal chandelier in his dining room. He made sure we knew they were his surgical tools. He hated fat, having had to cut through so much of it, so I wondered if he might have been doing his best to inspire loss of appetite. From where I sat at the opposite end of the massive, oval mahogany table, he seemed tiny standing behind the enormous bird while clasping his glistening blades, like a wizard who had lost or no longer needed his pointed hat.

I worked as his secretary, and general office assistant throughout my high school and early college summers. To this day I remember our peaceful lunches with fondness but also remember feeling very shy, somewhat distant and uncomfortable. I recall not being able to chew easily. I never discussed my desire to become a doctor with him, or anything personal.

I had no idea how he felt about women doctors, or how he would have felt about my ambition. I feared dismissal too much to risk finding out. He had so much power within our family that I feared he might even influence my father against me. Although my dad had supported my goal, I did not have much faith in his ability to evolve or maintain his own perspective on emotional or professional matters outside his own field.

He and Doctor had already fused together to fight any attempt on my part to enter religious life. They had written letters together to the superiors of religious orders, and to a spiritual director I visited monthly, whose approval would have been necessary for acceptance. They did everything they could to wipe out what I thought was my vocation. My father used Doctor's power to secure his point, and they were in complete agreement. They worked efficiently together, and I was told to forget religious life. Both felt I was using it to run away from the trauma of a difficult life. They were correct, of course!

During my second year at college, Doctor's hands were shaking too violently from Parkinson's to allow him to perform surgery, and he retired. By the time my father died and Ellen and I had become Babe's children, he was dying. I was left to attempt communication with Babe who would immediately call Nonie to help with any and all decisions. On one occasion Babe went into the kitchen to call Nonie following some intense conversation with Ellen, and lifted the phone off the wall.

"Decisions, decision, decisions," chirped Ellen playfully as she removed the phone from Babe's hand and replaced it into its receiver.

Ellen could do things like that, but I couldn't fight the phone verdict, not while grieving for my father, and not without him.

Babe and Nonie encouraged me to join the teaching profession as they had done. They believed it was a good profession for a woman.

I felt locked into a clearly defined girlplace. I had no fight in me. I was the unworthy one who so deserved to be beaten that people on the streets didn't even notice. I was the guilty one who had cost my father his freedom. I was the grieving one who had lost my closest friend.

Get Married

Fantasies of married life did not dance through my strained mind as I anticipated finishing up what was left of college. I believed my troubles were behind me. I had survived my father's death, my mother was locked away, and my sister and I had a new family as Babe's children. However, I knew I was expected to become a teacher, oh, and get married.

Get married. I sure didn't know much about marriage. My mother and father had slept in separate rooms when they were in the same house. The nuns and priests, though tender and affectionate, knew nothing about it. Throughout my entire life I had never witnessed any level of intimate romantic expression. Although without constructive role models, I hadn't destructive ones either. I missed out on the dirt, shame, and secrecy so lavishly sprinkled on sexuality for so many.

Sure, my aunt Babe had done her maidenly best to tell me about sex. I was twelve when she believed I should know these facts for my protection. Perhaps she'd noticed my infatuation with my eighteen-year-old piano teacher, and this was the basis for her concern. She told me I could learn more on the subject by talking to Nonie because her sister was a married woman. Never comfortable talking to Nonie about much of anything, I took a pass on that suggestion. I thought the new information was really disgusting. Since I'd never had pets, visited zoos or lived on a farm, my understanding of reproductive behavior suddenly depended entirely on Babe's lecture. I had believed until this moment that a woman said a prayer and then God gave a baby if it was His Will. I loved babies, so my reaction to this knowledge was to figure that whatever a soul had to do for a baby, a soul had to do.

Soon after Babe's simple plumbing lesson came the forbidden disclosure of my father's homecoming to greet my appearance. Added to guilt for my arrival into this world came shock; he'd engaged in such a pipefitting. I couldn't picture my parents within feet of each other.

By the time I was a college student I had discovered that my human body could become aroused, and had once traveled to a different borough of New York City to confess the horrid sin of masturbation. How terrible, I believed, to defile the locus of God's relationship to the Church. What I had learned about the meaning of sex was almost entirely symbolic. This attempt to live a symbol and deny sex its rightful biological reality led to unresolved craziness and abuse for myself, and I believe for many locked into cultural symbols as reality. I had been warned that masturbation was not only a sin but also a mortal sin. Mortal sins were the serious ones that could throw a person in hell should they die before getting to confession. So death while masturbating would impose a wake up in hell. Imagine!

Open, natural discussion on the subject does not take place for many children, even today. Recently, while giving a lecture to Catholic educators on sexuality, I expressed my hope that adults no longer taught teenagers masturbation was sinful. There was a stunned silence in the room as if they'd heard gunfire. The group could not cope with this subject, though all were supposedly mature adults. Obviously these grownups would not be able to talk spontaneously with children, even their own. Without self-acceptance we cannot give acceptance to others, a truth for all facets of our common humanity.

Sex that symbolizes Christ's relationship to the Church or the giving of an entire selfhood is far removed from the release of sexual tension. Sex as symbol fosters an unreality in danger of divorcing believers from human personality. But sadly, when persons rebel and give up on the symbolism, sex often becomes a means of exploitation, control and domination. When exploitive persons are referred to as animals, it is an injustice to our furry friends who employ sex for species-specific mating dances. Lost in all the confusion is awareness that the gift of sexuality is enjoyed most when used as a tool to express human love. But then, engaging in conversation and enjoying a meal are also most enjoyable when experienced within relationship.

Relationship? Unfortunately as we enter the twenty-first century there is more understanding about sexual functioning or lack thereof than there is awareness regarding what constitutes comfortable relationship. And the communicative skills required to maintain satisfying relationship too often seem mysterious.

The intricacies of wholesome sexual relationship were beyond my college-day comprehension. Awareness of my biology did not teach me anything about using sexuality to communicate feeling. I was too traumatized to feel much anyway, and my understanding of love related only to God.

When children relate to adults who accept and enjoy their sexuality, they learn the outward signs of health and the subtle dynamics that indicate the enjoyment of attraction. This does not mean they witness or are exposed to seduction or disturbing adult behavior.

During the sixties we used to speak about good vibes. Some today speak of a healing karma. Hard to define, and yet awareness of the subtlety within human relationship makes all the difference in being able to engage in satisfying relationship. My lack of awareness stemmed from a lack of role models, but for others there might be some neurological block to perceiving these subtleties.

With the exception of a few novels, I obtained some glimpse of interpersonal dynamics through the Metropolitan Opera Company. Taking advantage of the fifty-cent, standing-room tickets, I soaked up as much opera as possible. The rich melodic music swelled my emotions, and New York City presented some of the world's best voices. Sexual desire portrayed on the stage never seemed to do anyone much good, but the theatrical dynamics were exciting. Therefore, the first guy I really liked knew tons about opera. Though a brilliant and fun friend, my relationship to him had about as much reality as an opera. But by the time my father was dying I didn't even have the energy for opera.

Within months of his death I met both Bill and Daniel. They had been friends for over a year, and were both members of the Young Christian Student organization. They, along with a group of other dedicated students, including some of my college friends, had lived together in Chicago the previous summer. Two of these friends spoke so much about Daniel's brilliant talents that I felt awed by and inferior to him before we'd ever met.

After I had finished taking the Government Census, I met Bill while attending a YCS meeting with some of these friends. He later told me he'd liked how I defined things when I'd spoken at this meeting, and so had looked me up. This took some effort, since he lived in New Jersey and knew little about the city.

About three years older than I, he was not like anyone I had ever met. His strong hands had a wonderful ease as he worked with wood, and I loved to watch them. At such moments he'd remind me of the many religious pictures I'd seen of St. Joseph the Carpenter. He was practical and aware of the problems of the earth. We sat on benches along the East River and watched boats, the Brooklyn Bridge and the Sky. He taught me about thunder and lightning in ways I'd never understood them. He didn't like to spend money, so we ate bananas in Central Park, yet he did take me to see *West Side Story*. He was an engineering student, but was about to take a year off to study liberal arts in Vienna. He departed after I had known him for six weeks, and we promised to write.

Then I met Daniel who had been away from the United States

studying in South America. Over a year younger than I, he had soft brown eyes and a philosophical sense of humor like my father's. When I was a senior in college I attended my social functions with him. I enjoyed everything we did together and was completely comfortable with him.

I remember going to a dance, probably at Daniel's parish church, since I recall visiting with his parents afterwards. I was amazed that I did not have to think where to put my feet, yet did not lead and did not follow. I became overwhelmed with so much feeling, so much tenderness that even my fingertips hurt. I got scared, really scared.

Maybe I trembled because I was actually feeling, and had no context into which to put my feelings.

Maybe I trembled because I was a coward, afraid he'd die. Not very long after I'd met Daniel he'd had tumors removed from his cheeks. I heard all about how miserable he was and how much pain he was in, lying there with his mouth open as the damn surgery drained. I shivered. Still picturing my father in the hospital, I never visited Daniel there. Perhaps I feared that if I dared love him I might lose him to death, as I had lost my father. Conflicted between a vague desire to hold him and a vague feeling I should run away, my feelings reflected the emotional paralysis that permeated my entire life. This had nothing to do with Bill. I could have written him about my love for his friend, and we would have remained friends.

To protect myself, and from an obscured need to protect Daniel, I started to serve his best interest as I imagined his best interest, without communicating anything to him. I projected my feelings for him onto a beautiful girl with long black hair whom I'd seen at that church dance. She was wearing a tight, dark dress and high heels. She was really thin, as I had never been. She would be more worthy of him. She was gorgeous. He so wanted to be a doctor, and I thought he should finish medical school before getting into the marriage-and-children thing. They were one and the same in our day. The beautiful girl with long black hair would be there for him when he was ready. Nice little opera I put him into, without asking him what he thought of his part.

He sent me this letter:

> "…there are times to smile and there are times to weep. I have not wept for two years. I feel I might almost be incapable. Yesterday coming back on the bus, this gal I'm very fond of, held my hand for a while. Only it wasn't my hand, not really …she felt compassion for me, and so she showed and showered me with all blessings except sex. So, at this moment, I thought I might cry—but not weep. Then as the ride continued, there was a graceful moment of her fingers and despite the fact that she did not move, she was no longer holding mankind's hand, but mine. And she became very aware of this, and she wanted to let go, for mankind's sake. But she didn't. She became a woman capable of speaking love in wombs and words and wanes.
>
> And so I've given you no description of this gal, but I hope some of the things I have said, have made her blossom before you, and if I've succeeded, then I am very happy, for this too is my joy. If I haven't then I shall smile, and say 'some day …'"

I don't believe I answered his letter. I think I just kept it to torture myself. I knew I had never given him a single graceful moment. I knew that. I didn't really understand that I didn't know how. The opera doesn't show you life that close up! A vague fear of danger and death plagued my spirit. Whenever I would think of Daniel, picture his many endearing expressions and almost feel his warmth, I would hear strains from the *Requiem* of Berlioz. Sometimes I would almost weep, but not quite. Beyond a point, I could not feel.

One evening Daniel, a few of our friends, and I visited his parents. He went off into the back rooms of his home and came forth with a very large oil painting he had completed. He rested its base on the kitchen table. He called it his *Bluegirl*. Interested in both medicine and art he had painted the beautiful, very ill child. Her disease produced an enlarged head with unusual features, and she was to become violent. She wore a blue dress. She had big blue eyes and a determined look. She had a hammer raised in her right hand and in her left she dangled a naked, fetus-like doll. She was poised to swing her hammer and destroy the forces that had created her...someday....

He was only about eighteen or nineteen and I about twenty, yet I know he noticed how awed I was by his painting, though I didn't say much. I felt more relationship to him through the nonverbal ways children communicate than through words, because I couldn't verbalize emotion.

After exchanging many interesting but non-romantic letters with Bill, and knitting him two sweaters, we became engaged by mail as he continued his studies in Vienna. I bought my own engagement ring and put it on my own finger. I traveled by train to New Jersey from New York City and introduced myself to his parents. Through our correspondence, we planned that he should finish his junior year of engineering in Pennsylvania, and I should teach for a year in New York City before tying the knot. It was an arranged marriage that we'd arranged ourselves.

When Bill returned from Vienna, now that we were engaged, he had to meet *The Mother*. Bill was the only friend I'd ever told about my mother's constant hospitalizations or the recent knife attack. Because he wanted to marry me, I decided this confidence was only fair. I never related my humiliation from our family violence, nor how much I missed my father. It was not that I kept secrets; I was just anesthetized.

We drove to the state hospital north of the city. The vague feelings of danger and the fear of death returned. After all, the last man I had brought near my mother had almost been killed. Her violent reactions were somehow my responsibility. I was burdened with fear and guilt for my family.

The half-conscious feeling of danger and death lifted as I approached the state hospital with Bill. He exuded a capacity for self-defense. He had been in the military for three years. He was not upset. He did not threaten my numbed self with emotions. Therefore, this bizarre adventure progressed in a matter-of-fact manner. When my

mother saw me from her barred window she hurled the most godawful, bloodcurdling screams. "Mary, Mary," came her resounding wails.
"Wow, listen to that weird one," exclaimed Bill.
"That's my mother!"

At some point a few weeks later, I can remember standing in my living room looking out over the East River. I had looked out over the river so many times from the kitchen when Daniel had called and read me poems by Auden or e. e. cummings. I confessed to myself that I was not emotionally in love with Bill though I loved and respected him. Through my love for Daniel I had achieved some sense of what it might mean to involve feelings with love.
As I watched the boats travel the River, I became aware of how much I loved Daniel. I sensed his childlike soul, now part of my own. I admired his dedication to medicine, my lost profession.
I felt his art, his music, and his poetry. I loved him.
And then my mind screeched to itself, "Forget that, Mary! Who are you, unworthy one with the dead and dangerous family, to consider such a thought? He has such loving parents. They've witnessed to you a kind of tenderness you've never even seen before. Would you want your mother to kill their only son who has so much potential to give the world? Forget—forget—forget. You are so ashamed of her. You are so afraid of her. Could you tolerate introducing him to her? Forget—forget—forget that for moments you knew you felt that other kind of love."

I may not have been able to bury this emotional awareness so deeply if I'd had some intimacy on which to hang it. Experiences capable of holding these feelings were beyond my imagination. My concept of soul kissing, for example, pictured souls mingling and rejoicing together within God if the lips of two people who loved each other touched. Soul mingling might bequeath many blessings but reproductive success is not one of them.
But there were more complex facets to this than I could

comprehend until years later when, as a therapist, I found them both interesting and heart wrenching.

I had blamed my need to protect Daniel on his illness, his younger age and gentle spirit. Sensitive to music, I'd felt the power in Beethoven's chords as I'd banged them out and softness in Daniel's tones as he'd played the *Moonlight Sonata*. I attributed this to my greater power, but perhaps it was only greater anger. Months earlier the need to protect Daniel had intensified after I'd visited his parent's to "bring them something of home" as Daniel had put it, while he was away. His dad had related the story of Daniel's birth, while his mom looked on adoringly. He'd been a small infant, a little over three pounds. There'd been complications, so he was his parent's only natural child. His father acted out his care for the little son as he told the story, pacing up and down their living room with his hands cupped. As Daniel's father gazed into his cupped hands I visualized tiny hands and feet coming up out of them. I'm sure the love emanating from those hands kept the tiny baby warm, and he lived. I believed he should not have survived to become subjected to the danger of my family.

And as I visualized those little hands and feet Daniel became a baby brother as the loving father relating the story of his child's birth became my father. He seemed so like my father, as both men were small, feisty, and had worked their way up from nothing. They even had similar small, square hands, and I knew my dad's hands so well from hours of playing chess. My father was still alive somehow, and through this devoted father I felt I glimpsed my daddy's love for me when I'd been born. Perhaps it wasn't all bad that he had returned to my mother for my birth. Maybe my existence had given him the joy I'd witnessed when listening to the saga of Daniel's arrival. And if I was such a joy to my father, maybe I wasn't so guilty for his suffering after all.

Years later, after my mother's death, it had to be after my mother's death, I visited Daniel's dad. We went hiking and out to dinner. Widowed, he cooked a fantastic dinner with vegetables from his garden. We watched TV peacefully as I'd done so often with my dad.

Following our farewell I drove to a supermarket parking lot and stopped the car. I wept uncontrollably until I could weep no more. Eventually I came to realize I'd finally wept for the dad I'd lost so many years earlier.

I had not wept when my father died. At that time college friends and professors had asked me if I'd loved him, when I returned to school so matter-of-factly following the funeral. Yes, grief can become frozen for decades. For me, my father lived until one fine day I was ready to weep and let him go.

With such father transference it is not surprising that I did not call Daniel, nor surprising I felt obligated to keep him safe. I thought of calling, but the telephone nauseated me. I struggled to overcome this disability when working as the US Census taker, but trembled each time I lifted the receiver. I'd picture my mother slumped in her pajamas with the phone in her hand, demanding something of someone or talking on and on. A phone was too aggressive for me. Girls shouldn't call boys anyway. I struggled to become my mother's opposite.

Bill would survive *The Mother*. I didn't have to worry about him. I decided I was lucky to have found a really good man who wanted to establish a family with me. That's what college-educated girls were supposed to do, and most had an engagement ring by junior year. College years were to craft interesting, supportive spouses and intelligent mothers, but had little professional relevance for a woman's personal benefit in most cases. This era might be difficult for many young women in modern North America to comprehend, but we were very liberated compared to young women struggling within cultures dominated by religious fundamentalism.

I was expected to program some eligible male to care for his offspring and for me because Babe had "no man in the house," and I no longer had a father. I determined the missing dimension of emotional love, to the degree I'd gained any feeling for it, wasn't important enough to talk about. After all, what was it in the light of eternity? These bodies were only going to die. I had almost died twice myself before I was seven years old. Bill would be a good father. I never mentioned my misgivings to Bill. He was not left free to respond to my reservations.

Bill's mother had many qualms regarding our upcoming marriage. She wrote a number of letters to me expressing her concern that I had not known Bill long enough. She believed I did not know him. Also, she was afraid I would lament marrying into a materially simple family. Although she was not afraid I was stealing her son, she considered me more upper class and feared that if I married him it would leave me with many unsatisfied worldly needs. Of course, from my perspective, any family that could behave non-violently had more status than mine. I always answered her letters with a kind of spacey idealism that offered thoughts about universal love. I'm sure my answers, such as the following letter, only fueled her concern.

June 21, 1961

Dear Mrs. Moeller,

If nothing is happening on July 4th I'd love to make it out to visit you on that day. I have been busy learning about teaching and watching my class for next year. They are very cute and very bright.

Do I know Bill? Though I know him, I would be dishonest to say I knew him perfectly. This, I see as a great blessing, for it allows us the constant joy of new discovery. I hope I never know him perfectly until eternity. Then, too, in considering the question of knowing people, we must also be honest and admit that there are many times we don't even understand ourselves. It would, therefore, hardly be surprising that we don't always understand others, even those close to us.

Bill, I suppose, could be confusing, as he is many-sided, yet he is one, as the only power motivating his steel will is his love for God. Bill's strength might be frightening if one did not see behind it his utter gentleness. Then, too, as far as I have known him, he is always himself. His honesty gives people a shock at first, as few are half so honest. But what constantly amazes me about him is that he has a vision few people have. There are many "religious people" who are concerned only with that which pertains directly to God, and there are many "sinners" who only concern themselves with human nature, but Bill is one of the few who sees that God made human nature beautiful and that it is only a weak will that decays the Nature Christ took to save men. Because he is a man, nothing that is human is foreign to him, yet all is directed to God. I am the human expression of his love for God as he is of mine. Since he is so many-sided and so strong it might be easy to complicate the point of this man's existence. He simply wants to use this life as an opportunity to love God through the human nature he now possesses. Everything else about him exists because of this fact. He wants nothing more from life but this opportunity, nor do I. Life is never a comedy nor a tragedy, but an opportunity, and Bill is doing his very best to take advantage of it. You certainly have a very wonderful and very unique son!

Hope to see you soon.

Love, Mary

Bill and I married in July 1962. His cousin was so shocked by the emotional flatness of our wedding that he questioned what was wrong, that Bill and I didn't even hold hands as we left the reception.

Yet I was peaceful, and loved my friend, Bill. With this good man I embarked on a journey to do good for our world. We shared a deeply religious value system. We asked those at our wedding to chant Psalm 127 with us; "If the Lord does not build the house in vain do its builders labor…" Perhaps we were more like the missionaries I had wanted to become.

Daniel was the best man at our wedding. The *Bluegirl* was his wedding gift. He had given her a wide wooden frame, and I was honored and happy to welcome her to our home. Eventually I would become afraid of her and hide her away, but at this time I hung her in our bedroom. She was part of the family.

After the wedding we moved to Pennsylvania where Bill was finishing his senior year at Villanova University. I taught fifth grade in an elementary school about an hour from home. Bill and I had been settled only a few months when Daniel, now in his first year of medical school, visited our apartment with a woman he said he was going to marry. She was not the girl with long black hair from the church dance hall. This was not in the distant future. I was in bed recovering from the flu and a miscarriage. Loss, loss, loss—a blanket of loss wrapped around me. Daniel sat on the side of my bed. I can still feel this gentle student seated there, holding my hands while defining my physical condition and his life. Some obscured feelings stirred, and I almost wept.

So life was to go on, ready or not. The lessons I had not learned would come back for resolution, as unlearned realities always keep lifting their heads for recognition.

New Life, Old Life

Bill and I had launched diligently into married life. After all, we desired to improve the planet. Following Bill's graduation from Villanova, we headed for the University of Connecticut where he enrolled in a Civil and Environmental Engineering graduate program. At the end of each academic school year we would travel to an area near the Rocky Mountain National Park where Bill and his doctoral advisor conducted research.

This professor owned land near the park that he was selling at an unbelievably low price. We bought five acres, and over the next few summers built an eight-room home in Colorado we called Summerhouse. During the school year we lived in a very small student apartment, but we'd already built our home for family connection and relaxation.

Near the beginning of his graduate studies, Bill assisted my return to college to try again to prepare for medicine. Biology was no problem. Chemistry earned me a huge breakage fee for knocking equipment off the lab table with my expectant stomach. And Bill patiently rolled balls all over the kitchen table trying to get physics through my pregnant brain. I accepted that medicine was not my destiny without a maid. The house would never be cleaned, and no one would eat. I obtained a masters degree in education instead, which Bill considered an insurance policy in case he died and I had to support the children. Babe and Nonie were pleased I'd become so sensible.

Despite his generosity towards my intellect, Bill was a rather domineering head of the house. A woman's place as Kirche, Küche, und Kinder (church, kitchen, and children) was part of his heritage. Marriage partners do not need differing skin tones to connect extremely different cultures. A dominant German male might be an opposite for the absent Irish father. Irish women of my day tended to be independent, even if taught subservience to men. I was even more independent than the usual Irish woman because I'd never told anyone where I was going when I took to the streets in New York City.

My childhood defense had been a flight defense, learned so well from my father. When Bill was aggressive towards me with either his impulsive temper or his dominance, I would become silent, cry, space out, or attempt to run in some way. I could not speak. Whenever he tried to teach me defense against himself, I perceived him as more aggressive, and I became more distant. For me, he started to become *The Mother*. More transference. With this unconscious identification, the terror I harbored contributed to my inability to defend myself in any healthy way. We began to spin around in a typical vicious circle. He became more frustrated at our lack of communication, and therefore, more demanding. I felt as if I'd be hit over the head with a two-by-four at any moment. I grew increasingly solicitous and fussed more over his needs than my own. To appease him, as I had tried to appease my mother, I became an ever more spacey second-class servant.

Unknown to Bill this vicious circle locked me into posttraumatic stress disorder rather than allowing me to move beyond it. I became deeply re-traumatized the very first summer we had traveled to Colorado. Our first baby was only a few months old. I had wrapped him and put him into his little bed near where Bill was working outdoors so he could watch over him easily. Our son was sleeping, and I told Bill I was going to walk down to the river, about a mile away. Today I would have worn a watch, would have told Bill exactly what time I expected to be back and returned at exactly that time.

When I returned, the baby was crying in his bed and I immediately lifted him. Bill then turned and saw me. He picked up a huge rock and held it above his head. He was a very tall man with extremely long arms.

With the rock held high he came running towards me screaming, "I'm going to kill you. I'm going to kill you."

I ran into the house with my son and slammed the door. Bill did not come in after me, but I was terrified. I was living with *The Mother*. I imagined leaving, but had nowhere I thought I could go. Babe and Nonie would not be happy to have me back. My sister was away at nursing school. Daniel was married and expecting his first child. I didn't want to bother any member of my very small family. It never entered my mind that I could become an independent person and raise a son, although I was a teacher.

It was not an easy time for Bill either, and by presenting his perspective I am not minimizing my situation or making excuses for him. I think it is too bad that persons can become so into their own defense and victimization, even when real, that there is no place for understanding the feelings of the other or others involved. So this is what happened from where Bill's feet touched the earth.

> Unknown to Mary, the baby had started to cry, and she was way later than I had expected. My anxiety about the situation increased rapidly. Mary, the city girl, was down in the canyon, somewhere, and I could not just drop everything and go looking for her. Eventually, with rising panic about her safety and in desperation, I bundled the baby and his bed into the car and drove down the dirt road to the river at the bottom of the canyon. I crossed the roaring white-water torrent on the narrow plank bridge and went to the end of the road, honking

the horn and stopping many times to try to call her above the background roar of the river. Having not been able to hear any response to the horn or frantic calls, and with rising panic about what to do next, I retraced my path back to the house. Oblivious to all the drama and trauma, Mary casually walked back and lifted the baby out of his bed. When I turned and saw her I totally lost it in a flood of conflicting emotions.

At the very least Bill and I should have been engaged immediately in marriage and family therapy, but it didn't exist. Only decades later did we understand and regret the trauma we had caused each other. Bill put it that our hidden raw spots had bumped into each other, as they would again and still can today, although presently we can claim our wounds and sometimes laugh.

It is easy to forget that concepts so common to our era were not part of general awareness during an earlier time. Learning-disabled children were called stupid or labeled retarded. There was no comprehension of ADHD. The damage done to children through violence or sexual abuse was not protected against or even acknowledged. And who ever heard of Asperger's syndrome? A psychiatrist friend of mine, who had known Bill for almost forty years, told me about this brain organization when she suggested Bill might fit the category. It is because I have come to understand what she meant that I know my trauma could have been avoided if I had worn, and looked at, a watch.

Life went on. In total I suffered three miscarriages, and we had three beautiful children. Although I had almost slept through their conceptions I had wanted each of them. Birthing, nursing, and cuddling my babies started to connect me to a deep, unknown inner self. Although I was still numbed from my childhood experiences and the tendency of Bill's unpredictable anger to keep those memories before me, I was beginning to experience rich emotion for the first time in years.

During these years my sister, Ellen, graduated from Holy Child and completed nursing school. She came to stay with Bill, our first two children, and me after her graduation, until she found a good nursing position.

To have some inexpensive fun and introduce her to the pleasures of children, Bill and I dug out slides he had taken when I was about to deliver our first child. As a student family, we did not have much space in our apartment, let alone a proper screen for showing slides, so we pulled down our white living room shades and proceeded. In most of these pictures I was naked, and in a few I lay on our bed in a thin white chiffon gown. Then adorable little Eric was born, and we advanced to witness the nursing mother pictures.

The next day I was on my way to the community laundry in our student-housing complex. I learned that our neighbors had gathered on the opposite side of the white shades, and watched the show!

In the years to come Ellen married a businessman and remained in Connecticut. They had five children, with their oldest child the age of our youngest. Although the children became close as adults, they were otherwise off-balance, in age, to form friendships as children.

Our youngest child was born. As the day for his arrival approached, I felt a passionate desire to experience childbirth without drugs. My obstetrician allowed this, although not common practice in those days. As my son's nose came out for air, I sat up on the delivery room table to greet his face, caught him, and then slid him out into our world myself. Probably because it was an easy labor and a third child, I experienced this as a mystical ecstasy integrating the human and divine. There he was, a new human person with huge hands and feet. His big eyes looked all around as if trying to define his surroundings.

I loved my babies. I loved kissing their little tummies, their fat cheeks, their fingers and toes, and even their snotty little noses. I loved the little things they said, and the funny things they did. Being subservient to their needs was so rewarding.

But delighting in little ones was not able to counteract the stress of my life. A few months after the birth of this son, my mind took off on a trip in search of answers. Oh yes, it could be blamed on postpartum hormones, an undiagnosed thyroid condition, and the fact that Bill had been away for a number of months in South America finishing his doctoral research. This had left me with the care of three small children, and care of *The Mother*.

It had been a big shock to Ellen and me that she'd been released from the hospital, since we'd been told at the time of her last knife attack we'd be safe from her violence for life. However, the rules changed, and she was returned to society. Bill and I found an apartment for her a few miles away in our university town. She could not manage unattended. Of course, that heightened my level of anxiety. Not only did I again need to defend myself from her real or imagined attacks, I had to assure that she did not hurt my children.

Persons who knew us at the time picked their favorite stress to blame. Funny thing, when you don't or can't define yourself, others are always ready to do it for you. Babe and Nonie were angry Bill had traveled so far away and came to help me during his absence. They were fantastic with the two older children, but they aggravated me because they continuously poked fun at my breast-feeding. Although I knew this was innocent, it was irritating, because they knew nothing about nursing or how important this special relationship to my baby was to me. After a brief stay they went back to Manhattan.

By the time Bill returned from South America I had started to lose my usual level of coherence. Soon thereafter, he arrived home from a day at the university to find I had lit about twenty candles. I was praying with the children to rid evil and ignorance from the world. He blew out all the candles. He whisked the children away to a neighbor. He tried to talk to me, but I made no sense to him. He had been raised in a tradition of German rationalism, not Irish mysticism, and I was about as far from pure rationalism as anyone could get. He had always told others he had liked me initially because when I spoke I made so much sense. He had always said he admired what he found to be my ability to define and synthesize. Now I was incomprehensible to him. It must have been terrifying.

He left his handprint on my face and threw me across the dining room, I presume to knock some sense into me. Once again he became *The Mother,* big time! I had usually been able to get away from my mother as an older child, but now I had no place to go. Bill became the devil to me. How easily we can make devils of each other!

Bill called the police and took me off to a hospital. I signed myself in to get away from him, though I don't think I really knew where I was. A doctor who cared for me wrote this poem and mailed it to my home about a week later, by which time I had signed myself back out. She called it A *Touch of Grace,* and her signature, "Lynne," is all I know about her.

> You reach out your hand for mine.
> Your grasp is forceful
> and shakes me out of my busy frame of mind.
> I look at you directly, hoping to catch
> A glimpse of who indeed you really are.
> And you return my unspoken asking
> With such a wealth of feeling
> our surroundings fade into unimportance.
> Your grip seems an invitation, even a demand,
> to stay with you awhile as you journey
> through realms few of us dare to go.
> Your hands express fear and searching,
> your face uncertainty;
> yet you seem so acutely aware of some level of being and existence
> beyond my own experience.
> We speak of the bridge our hands have formed,
> Of you as you and me as me.
> You give me an awareness of the depth of meaning of the words
> "separateness" and "togetherness" that is rare and unique.
> Simultaneously you convince me of our
> very human needs to be each his own individual self
> and still to touch one another with sensitivity and firmness.
> Through our meeting you have helped me
> learn something of the art of communion person to person,
> A very beautiful gift. My thanks.

Another doctor, a much more clinical person, spoke with me about divorce. I should get one, he felt, because I was an abused woman with my face smacked and a side that was black and blue.

No. Bill was a good man and didn't deserve to be dumped. I had really frightened him. He could be impulsive but never malicious. Maybe the lack of any premeditated malice was what had captured my father's compassion when he'd speak of my mother as "basically good." It is as if a well-intentioned person suddenly comes under the influence of an uncontrollable force. And when we become afraid and lose language, violence so easily erupts.

Today I understand more about the terror Bill experienced when I lost the verbal ability on which he depended. His relational eye contact had always been poor and his non-verbal communication almost non-existent. He didn't know anything about all those subtle ways humans interrelate. Since I was emotionally numb, and he may have Asperger's, our strengths resided with intellect, and we understood emotion or anything else through verbal discussion. My honesty and capacity for definition gave Bill a feeling of secure connection. He would never have married a game-playing wizard who manipulated others with words or actions. He has an uncanny sense which enables him to avoid such folks.

I don't deny that I had been stressed by all the vicissitudes of life others had listed as relevant to my trip into outer space. It was exhausting to be alone with three little ones and a demanding, difficult mother. Yet I knew within myself that the big stressing factor was simply my level of sexual attraction for my obstetrician. I had never dealt with such feelings without repressing them. Now I felt their full force. I really didn't know what to do with them. Because they caused me a great deal of conflict, I tried to spiritualize them. After all, I'd always put every other feeling into some kind of religious context.

Perhaps concerned gynecologists should receive more training in psychology unless they want to make arousing the erotic potential of women part of their job description, which could be harmless if they did not take it personally. Unfortunately, my doctor had taken it personally, adding to the stress of my life. There is an undeniable physical relationship between doctor and woman. I delivered three babies into the hands of this warm, charming guy, and through the experience of relaxed touch had broken the frigidity I'd locked into in relationship to my lonely father. I felt very safe and relaxed with him. He was there during the wondrous experience of my last child's birth. When the anesthesiologist made his usual appearance, my doctor sent him away.

"She's going to do this her way," he said with eyes smiling above his mask.

Husbands were not allowed into our hospital's delivery room at this point in time, so the doctor was with me for my great experience, not Bill.

With feelings so out of rhythm with any prior experience or religious dogmatism, I now began a process of questioning and redefining my belief system. Over the next few years I read many books and talked with different kinds of people. All those who had taught me how I should perceive the world seemed to cancel each other out. I studied animal behavior, and through this study I began to remove religious symbolism from sexual behavior. Sex was sex to animals. It seemed more honest. Neither the virtue of fidelity nor Christ's relationship to the Church remained associated with sex for me any longer. I came to the conclusion that when love was the motivation it did not matter how love was communicated. And acceptance of birth control with the advent of the Pill separated sex from conception. Sex could now become a tool for the communication of love. I did not believe sex and love were the same reality. Love was still the Light, the heart of God. I simply saw no reason why sex couldn't be another expressive tool. Never having been abused sexually, I had nothing against sex, as do those who have been abused, shamed, or taught about it from the gutter.

This personal inquiry took place during the late sixties and early seventies when everyone seemed to be questioning everything anyway. I sure fit right in. The spirit of this hippie era allowed me the freedom to evolve through the adolescence I had never had.

My concept of the erotic was still totally intellectual. On an experiential level, I was a moron. Whatever curiosity I had about the subject was put aside when Bill completed his doctoral studies and took a teaching position in Florida. Packing three small children and a household to relocate at the southern end of the East Coast required that practical considerations take priority. My mother had been moved to an apartment near Ellen's family in Connecticut. Since she had been blamed for my stress-out, she was sent to stress out my sister.

I was not impressed with Florida. Far away from New York City I felt ripped from everything I had ever known. My eyes scanned the new environment and discovered only endless flat grids filled with boxes sporting trees like little green umbrellas. I found no shade from a New England maple tree or a gently swaying oak. Most months were too hot and humid for me to play outdoors with the children.

On one such blistering day I became totally fed up with my long, thick hair falling into a poopie diaper. This was the last time that was going to happen, I decided. Hiring a sitter to watch the children, I went off to have my hair cut short.

When Bill came home from work he asked, "Where is your hair?"

I told him I'd had it cut, while looking rather incredulous because I thought that was obvious.

"*Where* is your hair?" he demanded in a louder tone.

I directed him to the location of the hairdresser, and he left, soon to return with my hair. Holding up a long, auburn ponytail, which had been carefully fastened, he looked triumphant.

"See, as I knew, they were about to sell it."

I was not sure what I was supposed to do with it.

When Daniel and his family moved near us to complete his advanced residency, it felt as if we had family nearby. He and his spouse had welcomed four children in less time than we'd had three. She was a great cook, and we celebrated often. Each of the seven children found a playmate near his or her age.

Life went on with lots of fun trips to museums and the beach, while my capacity to communicate any feeling, even anger within a loving relationship, remained dormant.

A year later Bill obtained a professorship as an engineer in Lowell, Massachusetts. Daniel and his family took care of our children while we went to make living arrangements. When we moved I was not sorry to leave Florida but was very sorry to leave Daniel's family. I was also sorry to leave our neighbors across the street. I fear we humans continuously disrupt community more than we were designed to disrupt community. As much as I disliked the hot, humid, flat environment, I had been content.

Onward

Once settled in Massachusetts, we discovered a town so small it is still governed by a town meeting, although only an hour from Boston. With the same energy and diligence mobilized to build Summerhouse, Bill now designed and constructed Winterhouse on a hill overlooking our little country road and a beautiful, farmed field. There was lots of room for our family and for others we might welcome.

The children were doing well in school and had made new friends. Bill enjoyed his work, and I became challenged by my teaching position in a private school for mentally handicapped children. Our family might have evolved along traditional lines, but I was no longer content. Feeling unidentified as a person other than as a solicitous servant, and confused about sexuality, I began searching for my relational self.

As far as I'd gotten, relational sexuality meant childbirth. I had cherished caressing the humans within me. Birthing had been a mystical experience for me, although some may laugh at such a notion. With childbirth at the center of my awareness I naturally recalled the unresolved feelings for my former physician who had been with me through these experiences. When I wrote to him explaining I'd removed my churchy symbolism from sex, he called and invited me to meet him in a Boston hotel. But once there, he could not function. Attempting to love I probably reached for him as for an infant, symbolically desiring to return him to the womb for rebirth. Perhaps the manhood of most men would pale if forced into comparison with a whole baby. I may have wiped him out. On the other hand, not everything that happens is my fault. His unexpected condition upset him, and I added to his confusion by telling him it didn't matter because love was all that mattered.

"Do you understand yourself?" he asked. " And where did you tell Bill you were going?"

When he learned Bill knew where I was, he almost seemed to panic, and we were checked out very quickly thereafter. I never saw him again.

Although I no longer symbolized fidelity with sex, I maintained a deep sense of fidelity. To be faithful to Bill meant I would always be honest with Bill. He had no tolerance for dishonesty and would always need to know where I was and the time I'd be back. He could have called me at the hotel to see how things were going if he'd wanted. And if I were going to be late, I'd call.

In the midst of a present day conservative backlash it may be hard to believe Bill and I were ever married. Yet even today every couple that survives describes what marriage is for them and defines the parameters of a distinct relationship. Each couple is unique, while all learn to bestow greater honesty, acceptance, freedom and kindness.

The era during which I searched for self-awareness was the very era the present day conservative backlash seems to be reacting against. We swing back and forth between extremes because discernment is so difficult.

For some, the sixties led to an exploitation of sex along with the openness to human sexuality. I believe that persons who have experienced intimate relationship will have little use for exploitive sex, and would even run from it should they have the freedom to do so. But there is often so little human connection in the lives of so many. They are then left vulnerable to buy into a belief that sex is the way to the connection most people desire. It is certainly advertised as the way to fulfilling human connection! I firmly believe that we need to teach young people by word and experience to identify the factors necessary for an intimate, human relationship. Once learned, the sex factor is much more likely to fall into a wholesome place naturally. But there is a huge lack of competent teachers!

Unfortunately, during these still controversial hippie decades, instead of respecting legitimate authority while questioning and possibly transcending it, too frequently there was a violent disrespect for all authority. Today we often experience a rigid authoritarianism. To respect an elder's outlook while disagreeing and presenting a challenging view takes maturity beyond that of many persons. Once again, there is a teacher shortage.

Someday we will swing back to find what was best about the sixties and seventies. There were good things happening during these years though much became confused and distorted. Make love not war. Not a bad idea.

Because this period invited my freedom to grow up, I persisted in trying to love men with a maternal, mystical sexuality. The males on the receiving side interpreted me as some kind of tease. I learned they had words for the kind of woman they thought I was.

Yet, I looked disparagingly on interpersonal sex that seemed to have orgasm as the motivating drive. Another person should not be used as a self-serving tension release with about as much relational relevance as a good sneeze. I fumbled on, probing for some undefined holistic love, and hurting myself in the process.

At some point I became open-minded enough to realize that the sexual communication of love by a man would have to move through the gifts of his biology, not mine. He had no place to house little ones within him. He could not catch and caress tiny feet tickling inside. What would sex be like experienced by one with an organ a hundred times bigger than a clitoris, and breasts a hundred times smaller than mine? Perhaps a man could not separate the drive for orgasm from a desire for unity as naturally as a woman, who uses this separation to nurture children. Only he would be able to tell me, which meant I would have to listen.

But to listen, I would need to feel totally safe and completely comfortable.

I didn't realize that level of security until I had been introduced to Steven through colleagues at the school where I taught. He became my friend, which created a safety zone. At this time my level of physical defensiveness and emotional numbness was unknown to me, yet I was able to open a door within the shelter of intellect. By the time I was introduced to Steven I'd managed to re-victimize myself, this time by failing to communicate love to men interested in sex. It did not even dawn on me that I was trying to communicate this love-stuff to guys not the least bit interested in love. For me, all that really mattered was the love that reflected the love of God; that saw the face of Christ in everyone. I suppose I was lucky that only one man had become aggressively angry, and also lucky he'd walked away.

Then Steven's eyes touched my soul, and I responded to them. Perhaps because we were friends, and because he came from a very religious family, he eventually understood my spiritual-sexual orientation. Because I trusted him I was able to understand another physical approach to reality, and allow emotional love to integrate these opposite poles. Joyously I learned the ecstasy that can ignite when the erotic embraces within a field of love.

Did I fantasize being held by this man's beautiful eyes and running off into the sunset with him, attempting to leave the pain of my life behind? Sure I did.

It was a wholesome and thought-filled exercise to imagine escaping, as through it I realized I was already deeply committed. I felt how bonded I was to Bill's truly good self, to our common parenting, and even to the communities surrounding Summerhouse and Winterhouse. Although fidelity had become divorced from sex for me, it remained an important virtue. I was deeply grateful to Bill because he had left me free to grow up in whatever way I had to, without even understanding me.

And I felt bonded to Daniel and would not want to tell him I'd left my home. I had no conscious comprehension of why I felt that way. I simply needed to be faithful to my childhood soul, and it was in his hands.

My life had a history I could not abandon. A respect for personal history and loyalty to those who have been loved over time forms a foundation for community. When the bonds of human love are discarded in favor of superficial values and materialistic designs, we become a society of isolated, empty vessels. We cannot escape the past but are free to embrace it and use our history to appreciate the present and enrich the future. Although I had matured since I wrote to Bill's mother, he and I still shared our desire to bring God's love to our world. Although we suffered a limited emotional relationship in our unusual marriage, we shared an almost missionary spirit. Many marriages with far fewer problems than ours, fail, because there's no common value system. And beneficial to married life, I had learned to appreciate Bill as a man, and not a scary subway character. Sex now had value for me and was no longer something to endure.

I became able to experience a naturally and beautifully selfish moment during sex. I felt this belonged within a committed relationship because it was selfish, and so subject to greed. Throughout my life I had monitored my greed for power, for material things, and for food. Now I acknowledged another avenue for greed. The energy expenditure required to indulge erotic greed is not a popular subject these days but then neither is consideration of the unfair use of the energy resources of the world.

I did not visit with Steven for a year as we secured a separateness, and I rejoiced when he, his beautiful significant other, Bill, our children, and I were all back around the kitchen table. One evening, following this distancing time, I became very angry at Steven about some little thing. I took my drinking glass and threw it against a wall.

Then I started to sob and began to pick up the hundreds of shattered pieces.

"We grew up a lot together," he almost whispered very gently.

Then I cried very hard. I had become really angry, expressed it without being perfectly rational, and it was okay. That was a first. And I had not even thrown the glass at his head, as *The Mother* would have done.

Over time my friendship with Steven improved my ability to communicate with Bill. As I had trudged along the path of personal growth, Bill believed he understood me, but felt I would never survive in this world without the protection of his dominating rationalism. He thought he saw things the way they were, and if I didn't understand the world as he did, then I did not perceive reality correctly. I had not been able to communicate when I differed with him, or anyone else, but attempted to appease anyway. I appeased *The Mother* in Bill and others. This continued to increase his frustration over our failed communication.

"I did not want to be appeased," says Bill today.

Steven encouraged me to speak, not truth, but my perspective. I admired his ability to define concepts and his precision with language, and struggled to improve my own. I became convinced no magic words existed to explain an idea perfectly, because another might have a different interpretation of the very words I used. There were no magic terms to assure another's agreement. I could only offer my world view attained through study, experience, and reflection, and respect that of others.

Recently a friend took Bill and me on an exclusive study tour at the Robert Mondavi Winery in California. After touring the vineyard we were taken to a cozy room and each seated before four wine glasses. Glass by glass was filled with a special wine and then we moved to a long, rectangular table edged with bowls of everything from various flowers and herbs to mud. With our wine in one hand we were to smell the various bowls and try to match the wine to the smells. From this experience we came to understand the Wine Aroma Wheel that determines whether a wine should be described as fruity or more like black pepper. The vineyard listens intently to the experiences of others to form a wine's description. I mentioned to our little group how often couples fought because they did not experience life the same way, and often did not have the same meanings for words used to describe their experiences, yet had no Wheel of Meanings to arrange these differences. As we were leaving many told me this was true for them. One woman wanted to create a Wheel of Meanings for her family's problem areas. It would seem the relativity of a grape experience is more defined and accepted than is the relativity of sexual, religious, or financial experience. Toast to that. Hail to the almighty grape.

Steven became a mediator between Bill and me. As a scientist and German himself, he understood Bill, and so could translate between our realities. As my success at communicating grew, Bill began to appreciate that my world view was my reality, and when it differed from his, he was not invalidated. We could differ and we could both be right. Eventually we were able to live the hymn we sang at our wedding, "If the Lord does not build the house they labor in vain that buildeth it." There was but one Absolute Reality in our home, because Bill and I accepted that our realities were limited by the diverse places our dissimilar feet touched earth. This unchained us to bow before the God beyond our perspectives.

When Bill's non-verbal language frightened or confused me Steven said, "Listen to what he says. That is what he wants you to understand. Do not interpret the non-verbal language."

As years passed this became a valuable insight. While living with my mother I had learned to pay concentrated attention to non-verbal language. Suddenly this talent, which I use as a therapist, was a hindrance to my marriage. Bill had been attracted to me because of my verbal language ability.

As he kindly edited this book he added, "I was not attracted to you because of your ability for nonverbal communication, which was largely unseen by me."

Steven helped me improve the verbal skills on which Bill depended, making my capacity for definition more precise.

When I studied Asperger's at twenty-first century conferences, I told Bill about the dependence on verbal rather than non-verbal language. He was excited, kind of relieved, and reminded me of the way Steven had told me to communicate with him. He had been exceedingly comforted someone had helped me understand his need long before recognition of this unique brain organization had emerged. He has explained to me that he understands emotion through verbal definition. That his verbal ability has tested in the genius range, unusual for an engineer, may reflect his dependence on language.

And I defined through Steven, and again during my instruction as a family therapist, that I had never been responsible for my mother's reactions, or anyone's but my own. My angers, jealousies, fears, loves became emotions I could choose to accept or reject. And because others were equally free to accept or reject their reactions, I was able to lift them from my shoulders. Should I set out to make another angry or fearful, for which lousy motivation I'd acquire guilt, the other's reaction would still not be my responsibility. I came to see the horrific blame-swinging guilt trips we can so viciously hurl at each other as but our frightened attempts to avoid personal accountability.

Learning the importance of forgiveness to nurturing the creative bond of human relationship may be vital, allowing progress without the destructiveness of bitterness and unremitting anger. Embracing forgiveness can help us accept that we'll be hurt and treated unfairly, as well as hurt others and treat them unfairly. We will all suffer loss, and no one will be able to improve on the past or remove death from the future. Death, the great equalizer, inspires humility, and humility helps us bend to forgive ourselves. Those who would rather be perfect, as only God is perfect, may pretend perfection, but it never works. Sometimes it is hard not to laugh at such arrogance, but that would not help anyone. Best to laugh with others and at ourselves frequently, because to live in a world without humor is to experience some form of hell.

I am very thankful for what we have. In this twenty-first century, persons can feel weighted down by descriptions of pathology so easily thrown around. There seem to be a million clinical diagnoses for every kink in the soul. Bill and I attempt to focus on our strengths, for it is our strength that has allowed us to embrace our tormented places. Through our soundness we could all hold hands and rise beyond the crippled children within our spirits, accepting them and thus diminishing their significance.

The fifteen years following my defining discussions with Steven were full and busy for the whole family. The kids were in the process of growing up within the best support and love we could provide. Summers were spent family-centered at Summerhouse. Bill and I worked industriously. He became department chairman, did some consulting, tended his beautiful gardens, and always had a woodworking project in hand. I had continued to teach mentally handicapped children and increasingly became involved with their entire families in the process, as coaching a handicapped child is certainly a family project.

Therefore, I was excited when I discovered the emerging discipline of family therapy and decided to join the profession. I graduated from Boston University with a doctorate, and went through years of internship and field training. Along the way, Bill and the children were often guinea pigs for various therapeutic projects and demonstrations. I am subject to teasing about some of them to this day.

Children are always watching and learning from us. They can tell when we are real and when we are trying to sell a fake image of ourselves. Sometimes they know our fears before we do and can feel our sorrow, joy, or confusion. Best to be honest with them and foster communication from the time they are small. When my daughter, Anita, was about nine, she started a book she called, *Watching Mother Grow Up*. This is an account of my personal evolution through her child-eyes.

> I suppose it all started in Massachusetts.
> Then, Mom was not very grown up, as you might put it. She used to sit around and chat to friends. Not that chatting is bad, but she would just talk for hours and hours, and it seemed

to me she never said anything.

I say again that I totally believe in talking because it would be very hard to communicate without it.

The reason why I say "it all started in Massachusetts," is because I can't remember very well before that. Because when we moved there I was only four.

So on it went like this. I would go to nursery school, my big brother would walk off to first grade, my dad would go to work and my mom and my little brother would stay home. My mom would chat or clean the house or something like that until one day she got a job.

The day my mom got a job I rushed outside to show all my friends the papers but they weren't really interested which made me feel terrible.

Well, it started out well enough. She made a lot of nice friends (one of whom she brought home to live with us).

By then we had moved to a real nice place in the country, a big house my dad had built. When we moved into our newly built house I was to start second grade, and I did.

My mom, as I said, started out fine. She got a real nice principal named Sam that she has had a lot of real nice fights with.

One day, after returning home from one of these real nice fights, Mom was all upset. I being-kind-of-not-supposed to be in the room when my mother told my father what had happened, hid in between the fridge and the dishwasher and heard the whole thing. Obviously my mom had had a fight (not a fistfight) with her principal (boss) but did not get fired and it turned out all right. Of course, I didn't think this way then because I was a shy little second grader, and I started to cry myself. Now, after a few more of these fights, Mom slowly began to stick up for herself a little. So soon enough Mom was fighting back to Sam and also to anyone else she disagreed with. And so out of what grown-ups call observational learning I started slowly sticking up for myself too. So off Mom goes talking back to Sam, and to my dad, who is about the loudest voiced person in the family and can also scare you half to death when he yells. She stood up to my big brother who THEN would do practically anything to get his own way.

Now me, myself, was afraid that my mom and dad would get separated or something with all these loud voices and stuff. But slowly and surely I would start to stand up to my brother. I still didn't dare stand up to my father, but I did understand that just because my mom and dad stood up to each other didn't mean we were going through a divorce.

Now, my mom just about had the idea but I was way behind. This I think was because both my mom and I learn best through experience. My mom could experience fighting with Sam. I could not. But I tried. I started to stand up to my best friend Beth but when I did she didn't understand and would think that I hated her. But I went on trying. One day I actually stood up to my dad. It went like this. My parent's friend Kathy was over but it was late in the night and my mom had gone to bed. Kathy was in the living room and my dad was at the kitchen table. As I said it was late at night and I couldn't sleep. So I decided that if I could listen to a *John Denver* record I would be able to fall asleep to it. I walked downstairs and into the kitchen and as soon as my dad saw me he started yelling at me for not being in bed and saying he had sent me there hours ago. But I decided not to cop out and run away crying. Instead I actually yelled back at him (with quite a few tears).
'All I wanted was to put on a record so I could fall asleep.'

Now I expected my dad to slap me over his knee but instead he sat me on his knee and said that he was sorry and that I could put on a record. All this time Kathy had been listening and later told me that she had cried herself because she thought it was beautiful.

I had had my experience so now I was just about caught up with my mom in that category.

What sponges children are! As I had watched my mother to determine the kind of person I did not want to become while adopting my father's coping skills, Anita learned as I progressed.

With lots of development behind us, a good financial situation, and stable work environments, we wanted to reach out with our lives to the disadvantaged, as had been our original mission. We adopted a child from South America. Our three children contributed their savings to this third world endeavor. The child was to have been younger than our youngest son, but she turned out to be older. She had been brutalized and abused beyond imagination. She trusted no one and never would. We also took on many foster children and runaway children. These were all children introduced to me while I worked as a family therapist for the courts. There was no place to put them as they had exhausted all options of the child protection system, so a judge would let or even ask me to take them home. Our experiences with children would be a story in itself. We learned that our feeble attempts at love couldn't fix everything if a child's circuits for tenderness had been destroyed by abuse.

I came to appreciate more than ever how fortunate my sister and I were to have had Babe. This knowledge has inspired a long-standing commitment to offer opportunity to young children. Every child needs someone to be there for him or her, to impart affection and to be worthy of trust.

By the spring of 1993, our own children and many foster children had launched their own lives. With more time available and a lot of experience behind me, I decided to open a private practice. My mother had been with us for almost two years and was doing well enough, and I thought a private practice would give me more control over my hours than did court work or university teaching. I maintained my commitment to those struggling to provide a good life for their children, and so planned to offer a generous sliding fee scale.

Bill and I decided to spend July and August in Colorado at *Summerhouse* before I was to begin advertising. We had made arrangements with my sister, our daughter and our son, to maintain my mother's schedule. She did best if we respected her routine and did not ask her to adapt to change. We were really grateful for this two-month rest, through which the mountains we know by name worked magic on our souls. The crisp air, the slow pace and ever-changing, wide-open sky had always helped us assimilate life's learning experiences. We had many friends and neighbors in Colorado we'd known for decades and it was refreshing to reconnect with them.

We drove home following our customary route, first visiting Bill's parents, then Daniel and his family, and finally Babe and Nonie in New York City. They lived together now in the large apartment that had belonged to Nonie and Doctor. We'd enjoyed a light meal with them and thought they were doing well, although Nonie, now eighty-seven, was very thin, and Babe, at ninety-four, shuffled along more noticeably. They hurried us on our way after lunch, but we'd thought nothing of it, believing they were concerned, as usual, for our safe travels.

Back home our family was happy to return responsibility for my mother. She was still able to manage her personal hygiene, get pleasure from her weekly shopping trip, and cook for herself. She liked to eat alone as she watched the six o'clock news.

Bill and I sat by our fireplace and raised champagne glasses in a toast to new beginnings. We were grateful for our safe return. We looked forward to another academic year and my new venture.

The phone rang. With a still half-full glass in hand I lifted the receiver.

Doctor's daughter informed me that Babe and Nonie were no longer managing well. Bill and I had just visited them. Perhaps they'd tricked us.

Babe and Nonie were experts at keeping up appearances because appearances were so important to them. Some thirty years earlier Bill and I had been severely reprimanded for carrying our firstborn up the stairs to the apartment wearing only a diaper, while transporting our clothes for the night in a pillowcase. We departed the following day with our belongings properly packed in suitcases. Nonie was ever concerned with what her neighbors would think. She was always in control of her world, and we had been in her world. Babe was really very easy going, but this was not her residence originally.

I promised to call them before I hung up the phone.

Suddenly the night had changed. We silently lifted the champagne glasses one last time and put them down on the glass table. The fire was growing dim. Bill, of course, had heard my half of the conversation and could guess the other.

He offered that we move them into our house for their last years. I felt astonished, almost speechless. We had just been celebrating a toast to our new life, free from any others living in the original structure of our home.

About all I could say was, "I think we should have some time to ourselves, finally."

Yet I knew whatever sanity Ellen and I grew up to possess we owed largely to Babe. I knew the sisters were a pair. I knew I would call them in the morning.

Answers to Prayers

Morning dawned. Whatever would I say to Babe and Nonie when I called? Bill's generous option offering our home was not an idea I relished.

So I rationalized. Suppose I did suggest it? They would appreciate the gesture and refuse to come. They were New Yorkers. They would not consider living in rural Massachusetts.

As an incurable New Yorker at heart myself, I had once struggled to fit into the rural landscape of our little town. I'd never seen a real cow, and there were cows in residence at either end of my street, lots of them. When driving, determining how to approach other cars on roads without a line down the middle had been a challenge. Out here, with woods all around, surrender to sleep was not accompanied by the screech of fire engines or the siren of an ever-needed ambulance. A chorus of coyotes would be the more likely lullaby. Neighbors never played their music too loud. There were no neighbors. No stone-faced towers with gaping orifices protected from wind and snow.

And although too infirm to attend Broadway plays or the Metropolitan Opera, Babe and Nonie would still want to sense their proximity. Never would they move to rural Massachusetts. Anyway, they'd assured me that when too old for independent living, all was readied for their entrance into the Mary Manning Walsh Nursing Home.

My generous soul decided to invite them to join us because they would never come.

So, I called them. It was a short call. They were not doing well at all.

"You are the answer to a prayer," Nonie exclaimed.

How, oh, how did I get to be the answer to a prayer? Whatever happened to Mary Manning Walsh? I never found out. I only know we began making arrangements for their move scheduled to follow the Christmas Holidays.

I had to prepare my mother for the arrival of her sisters-in-law.

My dad had never wanted anything sprung on her. He had always tried to give her time to adapt. When he was dying of cancer I thought he should tell her the truth. We went over the letter he was going to send from his hospital to hers, but that letter was not the one he mailed. He sent the following letter to my college address and explained:

> I wrote to Mommy today but in a general newsy way. Instead of writing the letter, the draft of which I had shown you, I decided to spread its contents over many letters and a period of time, depending on how much she presses the point. My reason for change of mind is that it was too forceful and since one must come to an understanding of reality from within nothing would be gained by trying to impose it from without.
>
> Mommy has many deficiencies that are hard to tolerate (being human) but she is an honest, sincere, kind and good person fundamentally.
>
> That trip to Holy Cross and back the same day seems like a long one to me but if you feel rested enough—go ahead and

have a nice time. Better not mention it to Mommy until you return. She has lots of time to worry.

Well that's all for now, Mary, so be good

Love, Daddy

Xoxoxoxo

This letter had troubled me. His insistence on calling my mother, "mommy," when I had never, never called her, "mommy," seemed some illusion on his part that ignored Ellen and my experience and suffering. Maybe it is very hard for a man to admit that his choice of a spouse gave his children a raw deal.

Then there was the incessant "don't tell her this," and "don't tell her that," stuff. This had permeated my childhood. *Pope Cornelius* had reality in his pocket and what of it could or should be disclosed was to remain in the hands of the supposedly sane. Such control over what another can or can't know, and such overwhelming assumption of responsibility for the reactions of another, undermines personhood and creates instability. But my father would not have understood anything of the sort, although today I'd love to try and discuss it with him. As do we all, he belonged to his era, and I trust his intentions were noble. He was a kind and good person. See—I sound like him. Perhaps almost all of us are kind and good, just controlling as hell.

My dad had been dying of cancer. That was just the way it was. Neither he nor my mother had the luxury of gradual adaptation to that reality.

Babe and Nonie were coming to live with my mother. That was just the way it was. Couldn't spread the news over time. Time would not give us forever.

So I told her Babe and Nonie were in bad shape and would be arriving.

She was not jealous that they would live in the original house with

Bill and me. She knew they did not smoke and that no smoke was allowed in there. She felt proud she owned much more space than they would have and expressed relief that she had her own place. She expressed some sorrow they had gotten so old.

"The end of life is always sad," she said.

She made sure I understood that their arrival into my home was not her doing. She actually wished me good luck.

I flew out of Boston the day before Thanksgiving to cook for them and discuss the final details of their transport. I still felt shock that this was really happening. I was in some quasi-state of disbelief. At least my psyche was not operating from subservience, but only from loyalty and obligation. I felt burdened.

By the time my flight landed, Nonie had taken a bad fall and been admitted to the hospital. Doctors reported she suffered some level of dementia, was incontinent, and a mystery to the hospital staff. They couldn't figure out exactly what was wrong and were performing a number of diagnostic tests. They felt she might have become overextended caring for her older sister.

When I arrived at the hospital Nonie looked very, very small in her bed propped up against pillows and covered up to her chin in white blankets. She was extremely thin and terribly weak. Occasionally her arms would start a strange trembling. When the shaking happened it kept her from being able to open her pocketbook or hold a drink. She told me I didn't know what I was taking on because she was very, very sick, had holes in her head and thought she should be placed in some corner to die.

The care of her older sister was paramount to her. They needed to be together. They had always been together. I told her I was honored to assist them and was so grateful for all they had done for Ellen and me. I expressed to her and to myself that everything would be just fine, then hurried back to Babe who was alone in their apartment.

A cleaning service had been keeping it spotless. The crystal chandelier was polished, the oriental rugs vacuumed, the beautiful art and furniture in good condition such that everything appeared as it had always appeared throughout my life. Babe was not spotless, however. She had always been a very clean and dignified person, and I found it sad to want to brush her hair, scrub her clothes and herself. Of course, I could do nothing of the sort. Babe was a respectable and reserved lady. She did not like to be touched. She did not want her long gray hair brushed. As long as she'd securely planted a neat, black-ribbon bow on top of her head, she thought she was groomed.

Early the following morning Babe shuffled her ninety-four-year-old body out to the kitchen, and we prepared Thanksgiving dinner together. She had always loved to cook, and enjoyed fresh vegetables, so she peeled a turnip. This was a major undertaking because, blind in one eye and with poor vision in the other, she had to feel her way around the thing.

She spoke of her sister and said she hoped the Lord would take Nonie rather than that she suffer on this earth. Babe wanted to be the one to die last because she felt Nonie was really dependent on her. Nonie had never lived alone as she had, when not caring for Ellen and me.

After dinner had been readied for later that day, I helped Babe to her TV and rest area next to her bathroom. When she was comfortable I left to take Nonie holiday greetings and some pie.

Coming up out of the subway at Columbus Circle on the West Side of Manhattan, I literally bumped into the Macy's Thanksgiving Day Parade. I had seen this parade many times as a child. Sometimes Ellen and I would watch it from a room in the Waldorf Astoria, donated for us by friends of my father who would do anything for his little darlings. In addition to enduring all the chaos in my family, I had experienced being indulged materially. Numerous home movies witness Christmas celebrations and birthday parties filled excessively with expensive toys and clothes. Maybe material goods were given as a peace offering for our lack of family peace. Peace and intimate love were never found packaged in all the stuff.

This day I stood on a sidewalk whipped by a freezing wind and watched as the Parade passed. I startled as a bloated float bumped into a street light post and broke it, causing fear and commotion among observers on the street below. Later, on the evening news, I learned a person had actually been hurt. There was no Waldorf Astoria for me this frigid day. There was no Daddy or Doctor to advise about the elderly sisters.

I moved beyond the Macy's Parade and continued to hike towards St. Luke's-Roosevelt Hospital on Tenth Avenue. I walked past the Paulist Church I had visited often as a young adult to hear the inspiring sermons given by these priests. On the steps of the church I saw a young woman with blond hair. She was wrapped in a white fluffy blanket, and held a cup in her hand. For a second I imagined her on a couch sipping a cup of coffee in her living room, wrapped in a furry white blanket. No, this was not a couch in a warm living room. These were cement steps. The lovely young woman held up her cup to a passerby, who passed by and went into the church. I thought of Nonie propped up in her bed, layered in her white blankets, and felt again some of the desire to serve that I had felt so long ago.

Turning back, I climbed those steps and spoke with the homeless woman. Once within the familiar church, I collapsed onto a pew from fatigue and disbelief. Was I really in New York City on such an overwhelming mission? I needed to rekindle the spirit of constructive service motivating me in the days I had pounded these same pavements desiring to be a doctor. I needed to sift out those inspiring feelings from the appeasing servant I had a propensity to become due to my own scars and insecurities.

As I half-knelt in the pew, my entire being sought love as a plant turns towards the sunlight. My mind floated as I placed myself into the embracing Presence of God and opened my entire being to Love. I felt every cell tremble and each nerve quiver to an inner music of exquisite tenderness.

"Help me, Love, bring Your love to this world as my envisioned doctor-self had longed to do. Help me surrender my own greed and extend myself outward, refusing to suck inward. Free me of devouring idolatries that my entirety can dance joyfully in freedom."

I sensed I was choosing to take care of Babe and Nonie, as I had once wanted to choose medicine. Conscious of personal choice, I felt control over my life and much happier as I left the church.

Nonie's pie finally made it to the hospital, and she said she'd save it for later. She was now hooked up to a heart monitor for twenty-four hours. She attempted to walk around with the little machine attached but was much too weak. Even thinner, she still talked about the holes in her head and how ill she was. The doctors could find little wrong with her.

I went back to Babe, and enjoyed Thanksgiving dinner. We really did enjoy our holiday dinner, because Babe loved to party and always wanted an excuse to celebrate. Even through tragedy, she found ways to laugh and revel in life.

During this Thanksgiving celebration she told me about my Irish immigrant grandparents and aware I might not have much time to get this history straight, I carefully took notes. Babe's real name was Margaret Donovan and there is a tombstone with this name on it somewhere in her father's hometown of Rosscarbery, Ireland. The original Margaret Donovan, her father's sister, had also been a teacher. She had died of "hasty consumption" at 32 years after crossing many dank bogs attempting to get Irish youth to go to school and learn. Her death devastated her little brother, my grandfather, Rikardus Cornelius. She had been tutoring him for the Trinity College exams when she died. After her death Ricky Con came to the United States. There he met Mary Driscoll, from Balinacarriga Castle, thirty miles from where he had grown up in Ireland. They married in All Saints Church at East 129th Street, on July 25, 1897. Remarkably, they had three children after their first child, a ten-pound boy, died during birth, supposedly destroying in the process my grandmother's ability to have any more children.

Within her community, Mary Driscoll was known to be very smart. Sick or injured people would bring their problems to her because she had a talent for fixing these medical difficulties. This immigrant population would only call a doctor for the deathly ill. My grandmother spoke and read Irish, as Gaelic was commonly called, and read the Irish newspaper to the blind and illiterate.

She was a very serious person with little use for frivolity. Thus she was described as getting very upset when her brother, Fluffy Driscoll, visited her family. Fluffy Driscoll was a beautiful dancer and a fun-loving character. He'd get the whole family up on their feet singing:

> One, two, three
> Balance with me
> You are a fairy, but you have your faults
> For the right leg is lazy, and the left leg is crazy
> But don't be Unazy
> I'll teach you to waltz.

Babe laughed and laughed at the memory of this dance. She spoke about how they wouldn't know how to respond to their small, round, golden-haired mother's proper seriousness. My grandfather, Ricky Con, was a much more playful person. He was also sensitive, poetic, tall and dark, with a prominent nose, like my father's and a rather long beard. One day, while he was walking back from a new store on the fringe of their All Saints Parish neighborhood, a group of young men picked up stones and hurled them at my grandfather. "Rabbi, Rabbi," they cried after him, as they threw more rocks.

I kept on writing until Babe was tired, and then I put my pad away for another day. I stood by as she shuffled to wash up and get herself to bed. Her shoulders were straight as she leaned lightly on her cane, but her feet never lifted from the ground. A holiday meant some extra wine, so her shuffle was even slower. Babe loved "just a little" wine.

"Put another wing on that bird," she'd love to say.

The next day I again settled Babe and headed for Manhattan. For a time I roamed my old hometown wondering when I'd ever see it again.

I walked the streets I knew so well, finally stopping at St. Francis Xavier Church on 34th Street to visit Father Frank with whom I had so often walked. He had remained stationed in New York City, so Bill and I would visit him whenever we could. One summer he had come to Summerhouse and enjoyed climbing the mountains. He had learned Spanish to communicate more meaningfully with his congregation, and many raggedy children ran into his arms when he called to them or they saw him. They conversed with him, and he tenderly answered them in their language. It seemed as if I had walked city streets with him for decades. For me, he was a Christ in the real world.

On this day, he said a Mass in a beautiful private chapel on 34th Street just for me. As I answered him with the response prayers I felt my link to the Church throughout the ages, though both saddened and angered by its injustices, prejudices, and abuses. He gave a gentle sermon detailing why he wasn't worried about my soul. Given that he knew lots about me through our years of dialogue, I felt warmed by his acceptance.

After Mass he said he wanted to accompany me to visit Nonie. It must have been to comfort me, because Babe and Nonie had never liked him too much, priest or not. Although *himself* was an Irishman, he loved to tease them. In his soft brogue he'd joke that they were LDI and not LCI. This meant they'd be "Low Down Irish" versus "Lace Curtain Irish." Babe, especially, would become infuriated. Her immigrant family had worked very hard to "make it" into the mainstream of society. She considered herself a professional, and Nonie had certainly married a professional. Material symbols of their success were important, particularly to Nonie. Frank was not impressed with lace curtains as he lived a life devoted to the low down. Humorously, he turned it all backwards, as he spoke with compassionate devotion about his warm, poverty-stricken friends.

Now on the way to visit Nonie, we headed for the nearby Sixth Avenue subway entrance. He got us really lost in the subways. He had always known the subways like his own name yet we went up and down steep stairways checking out trains, until I took charge and found the one headed towards the hospital. I was trying not to cry. My old friend was also old now. He, too, was losing it. He, too, was going to die.

Frank had always been there to encourage me, yet I needed to assure he would not get lost returning to his rectory after our visit with Nonie, and escorted him to the correct train. As I watched him limp away, bothered by an old injury from the Korean War, I almost wept for him, and for my dead daddy. I felt as alone as I had felt when I lost him. And I lost Frank a few years later from Alzheimer's disease.

I returned to continue my visit to Nonie without Frank, and so discovered the Hospital had decided Nonie must leave because the doctors couldn't find anything wrong with her. Although they hadn't discovered a particular problem, she continued to insist that she was very sick and had holes in her head.

She was extremely frail, and would not be able to walk up the steps to her apartment. She could barely walk at all. I consulted by phone with Bill and my sister Ellen. Babe hoped everyone would do whatever made life easiest and Nonie the most comfortable. Nonie wanted us aware of how ill she was and the burden she felt we were accepting.

We determined it would simplify the situation if we could settle Babe and Nonie once rather than twice. We decided to head directly for Massachusetts.

This decision gave Bill a few hours to plan for their arrival and buy any materials he might need to prepare a place for them. My action man spun into operation. Bill is a tall, thin person with long arms and legs. He is constant motion. He has an indefatigable capacity to perform efficiently in perpetual action until he decides to go to bed, whereupon he instantly falls asleep. So in just a day Bill constructed a wall complete with trim and paint that divided our large living room into two halves. This wall also contained a door that allowed passage between the sides of the sectioned room. Yet despite the short period of time, he installed this divider in such a way that one day it could be removed without showing any damage to the walls, floor or ceiling to which it was attached. Babe and Nonie's room would become the half next to a bathroom and near the kitchen. This set up would keep them on ground level. Then Bill rented a little truck and early Sunday morning came to New York City to pick up their beds, bureaus and clothes. The rest of the apartment would be left locked for some future venture.

I hired an ambulance for Sunday, brought Babe to the Hospital, and prepared to leave. Babe was stoical and calm while Nonie appeared frail and shaky. They were extremely happy to see each other as we entered Nonie's room. Nonie talked about how they would stay together, how they'd always stick together. Because she was tired, I found a wheelchair for Babe and the sisters held hands from their respective wheelchairs as we journeyed down an elevator to the ambulance. They smiled and looked angelic.

As we approached the ambulance the drivers came to help us. These two large, kind men seemed as if they could be at ease in any situation and certainly helped me feel more relaxed. Nonie was stretched out on a cot in the ambulance. Babe and I sat up along the side. Slowly, in dense traffic congestion, we left the settings of my youth. One attendant held a pot for Nonie to pee into many times during the trip. Babe and I stopped at rest areas along the way. She owned only slippers, or heels and stockings. My ever-perfect lady had on her heels and stockings. She would not wear slippers in public, so she teetered to the bathroom in open-toed shoes with the thin strap around the ankle. As had so often been the case during my life, hindsight produced clarity. I should have invested in a pair of travel shoes for Babe.

The normally five-hour trip took an endless eight hours. This was the Sunday of the Thanksgiving weekend. We were so stuck in traffic the siren would not have helped move us along.

Finally, we made it. Babe and Nonie entered our rural town, many miles from New York City. Bill and Ellen came out to greet the ambulance. Somehow, Bill was back and everything had been set up. He was cheerful, supportive, and efficient. He did not look tired after his endless construction and driving. I was exhausted. I have never been indefatigable! Bill and my sister made Babe and Nonie feel very secure and welcome.

The worn out drivers pulled Nonie from the ambulance on a stretcher. She was still trembling and very weak. They wrapped her in blankets. I went ahead to hold the doors.

There would be two sets of doors to open. When Bill constructed the apartment for my mother he built a common entryway to house both the door to the main house and a door to her apartment. The men each held an end of Nonie's stretcher and approached this enclosed space. As Nonie was brought into it, *The Mother* emerged from her doorway leaning on a cane. She looked down into Nonie's face and Nonie up into hers.

Nonie's expression seemed to scream, "Oh God, I forgot about her. She's here."

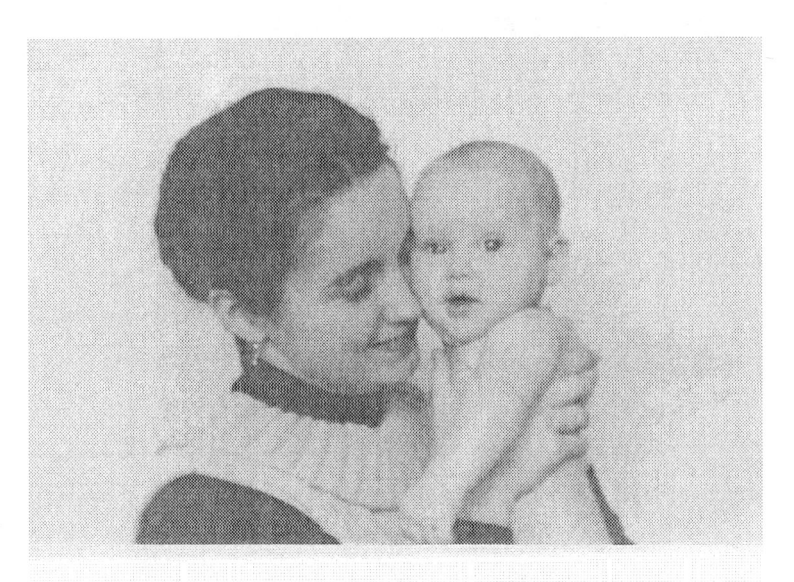

Anita and I 1966

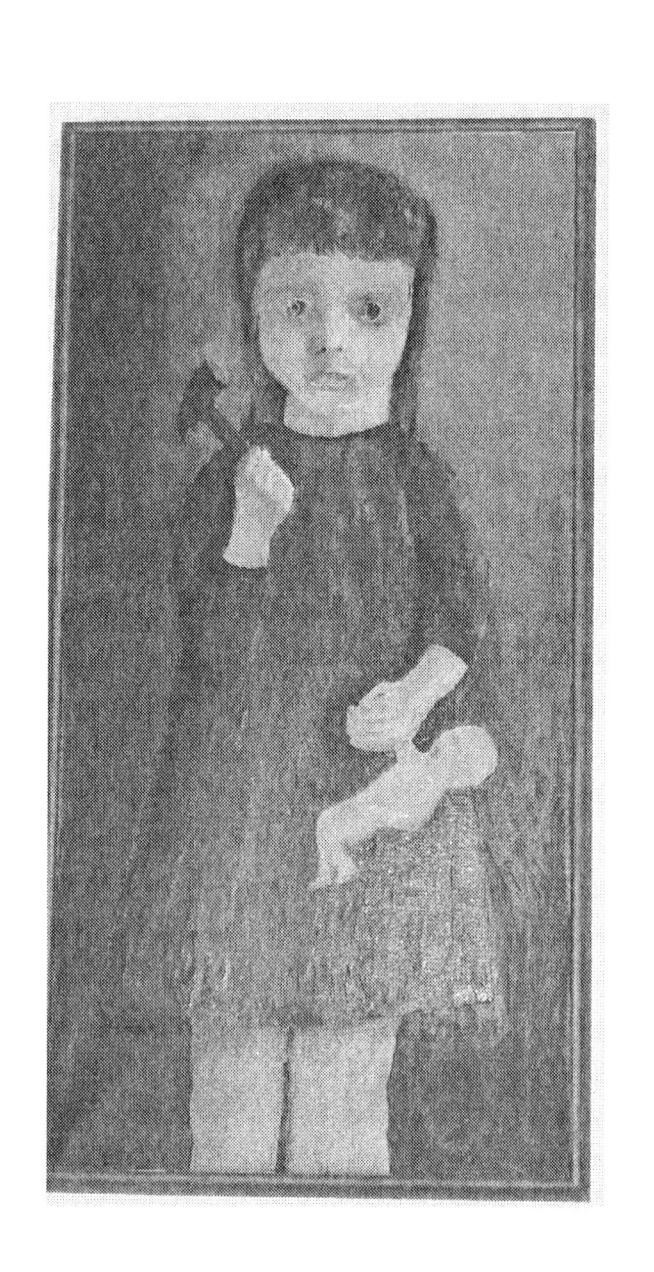

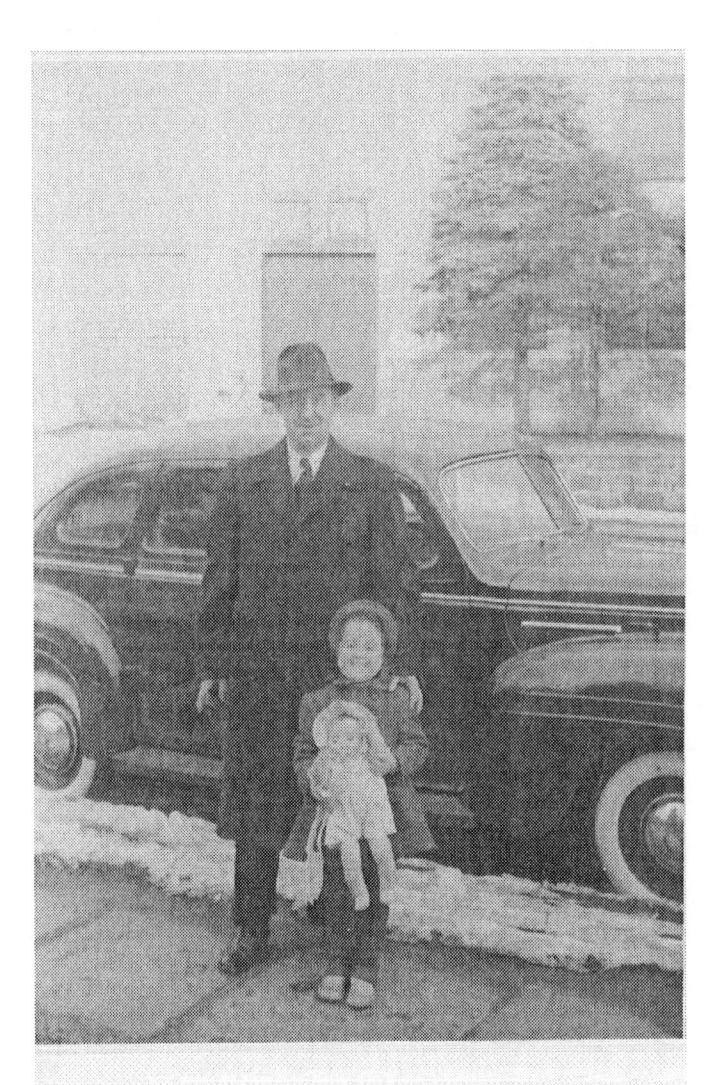

Dad and I 1942

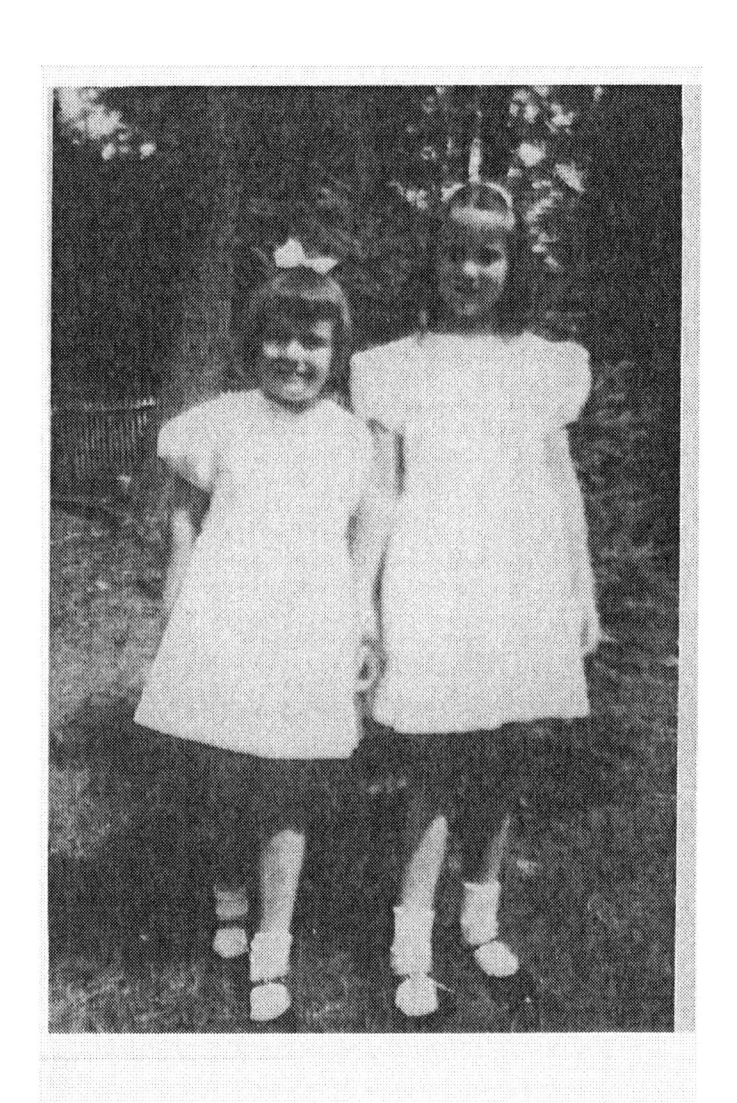

Ellen and I 1945

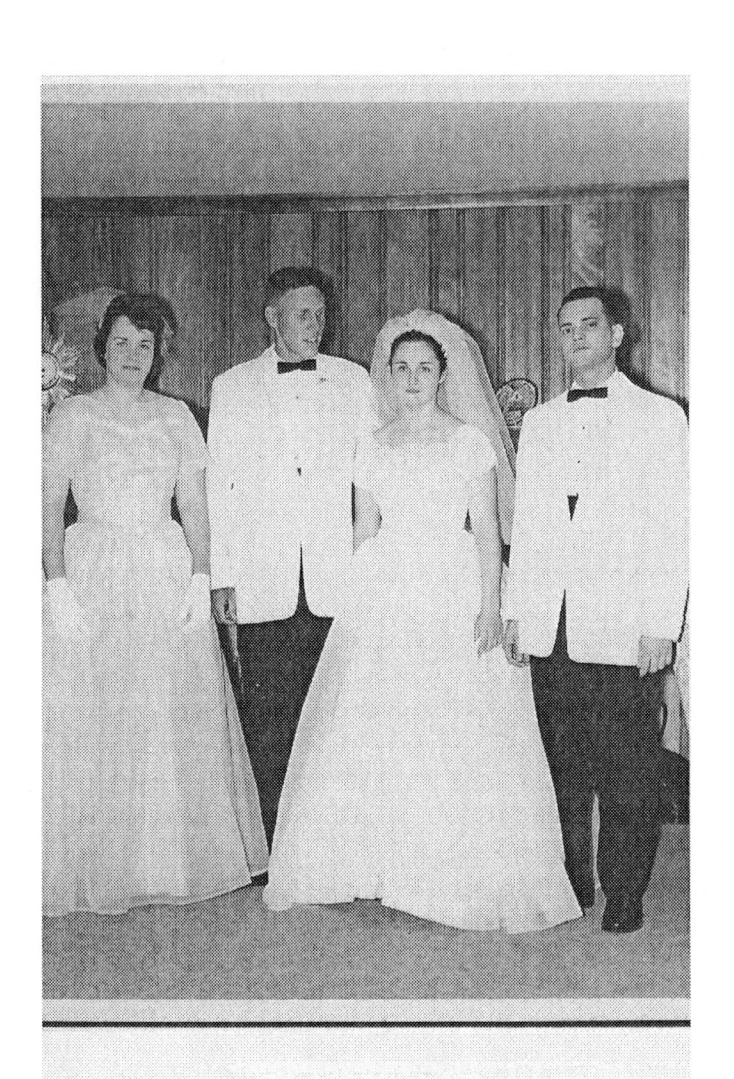

Ellen, Bill, Daniel and I 1962

All Together, Girls

They had not seen each other in years. After peering at Nonie *The Mother* glanced towards Babe who graciously managed to wave. Seemingly satisfied, my mother turned and headed back to her apartment.

The rest of us followed Nonie as the ambulance crew put her to bed. Ellen and I supported Babe who was extremely tired from the grueling trip. When Nonie was comfortable, Babe literally collapsed. We caught her as she began to slip towards the floor, and laid her in bed. She seemed semi-conscious but told us she was only tired and would sleep. Always a great sleeper she had taken a nap almost every afternoon during the years we'd lived together. Babe slept awhile and recovered, but months later when she was diagnosed with heart disease, we remembered this incident and were amazed she had survived the events of that day. Babe had a mission and was determined to settle Nonie in heaven before her own appearance at the pearly gates.

A local doctor and visiting nurses were expecting Babe and Nonie, although not for a few months. We had researched our local services to determine what would benefit everyone. Medicare allowed visiting nurse and home-health aide for the homebound. My mother did not qualify at this time because she was still able to shop, make medical appointments, and go out to lunch.

After an initial doctor visit, the nursing staff met with Babe and Nonie to set up a schedule for health checks and personal care. Nonie had no problem with home-health aides bathing and attending to her. She enjoyed this attention twice a week. Babe would have none of it. She allowed the accoutrements to be arranged so she could wash herself. The nurses reckoned this as the difference between a widow and a spinster. For whatever reason, Babe had never liked to be touched. Although a warm personality, she had never been a hugger. Even her greetings and farewells were somewhat stylized. Now, this aversion was making her cleanliness difficult to maintain and her long gray hair a problem to manage.

Nonie improved. We placed a portable potty-chair next to her bed so she could swing herself onto it and soon she no longer suffered embarrassing incontinence. Babe's bed and recliner were on the other side of the same large room, and at first she would turn away during Nonie's relief trips, but eventually ignored her or continued to watch television. Even in extreme old age we are adaptable, or perhaps those who reach advanced years must be adaptable. The doctor prescribed a little anxiety-reducing medication that facilitated Nonie's tranquility. She ate better. She strengthened, and soon she was able to walk to the bathroom on occasion, and to the kitchen to fix lunch for herself and her sister.

At daybreak they would shuffle out for breakfast. They started with coffee. Babe liked hers black while Nonie preferred some milk. They loved hot oatmeal, and as I stirred the pot on the stove they would chatter away as they had for decades. One morning they spoke to me about my grandmother, Mary Driscoll. Babe revealed how she had wanted to become a journalist but her mother had thought that was nonsense for a woman. She should be a teacher. Then Nonie said she'd told her mother she wanted to go into business, but her mother would hear none of it. The business world was for men. She should be a teacher. Babe obeyed her mother but confessed she would attempt to punish her by telling horror tales from teaching experiences. She wanted to show her mother journalism would not have been a bit more risqué. I listened and froze. They hadn't wanted to be teachers, and yet they had insisted I be a teacher? They had treated me the way their mother had treated them?

I looked over at these very old people who'd had so much power over me when I was a young woman desiring medical school. Suddenly I felt angry I had allowed them so much influence over me and incensed at my own powerlessness. I couldn't understand why I'd been unable to behave as the person I'd become. And couldn't they have rejoiced to see me go beyond where they had been trapped as I had celebrated the achievements of my children?

Then I recalled a visit to the old apartment with Bill years before. Our children were teens at that point, and I was enrolled at Boston University. I'd been telling Babe and Nonie about my studies as something to talk about and because I thought they might be interested until Nonie waved her hand that I be still.

Suddenly she shrieked, "You goddamn superwoman."

I'd felt really hurt.

Bill had been within hearing distance and still recalls Nonie's words and voice tone. I never mentioned my professional life to either Babe or Nonie again. In years to come, should I try to ease some situation within the family by drawing upon my knowledge as a therapist, my comments even when presented without psychobabble, were dismissed as irrelevant. I had never been conventional enough to suit Nonie. I'd always been too logical and independent for Babe.

"Mary," she called, "are we ever going to eat this morning?"

Oh yes, current realities were breakfast and oatmeal. Well, life is always only what it is. It was not the fault of these old gals that I hadn't been able to define my identity. I wondered if they remembered my desire to become a doctor, but decided not to ask. Perhaps I was afraid it would hurt too much if they had forgotten. But the past is there to be learned from and forgiven. It can only be forgiven because it can never be changed and real tragedy occurs when we try to escape its truth and hence become doomed to repetition. I reached within myself to embrace and forgive the fragile young woman who had been so easy to influence. After all, when I'd learned to walk and skip I had not deplored my days of expert crawling.

Although Nonie made great strides, she still talked about the holes in her head and how ill she was. She would only wear a cotton nightgown and a robe. She decided such garments were the kindest to her skin, and that her skin couldn't take any harshness or weight. She was focused on lists, all manner of lists. There was the list detailing who was to inherit what, the medication list, and the list of when her sister had bowel movements. She wrote down and went over her lists again and again.

Their wills were updated once Doctor's son-in-law sold the apartment. Business was all straightened out.

They signed living wills, and I was documented as their health care proxy. Neither Babe nor Nonie wanted extreme measures used to prolong their lives. They did not want feeding or breathing tubes, they did not want antibiotics, they did not want to be taken to a hospital, and they did not want pain. Therefore, pain medication would be okay.

It may be hard to talk about these things, but I imagined it more difficult to make decisions for them without having their clearly expressed thoughts comfortably lodged within my mind. It was a relief to know I was going to care for them in the way they wanted to be treated.

Babe did not understand why the visiting nurses came to monitor her blood pressure.

"I'm almost one hundred," she'd complain, "so why don't they go spend their time on the young?"

Babe liked only one nurse. When Sarah visited, all seemed to go well. She and Babe would laugh together and tell life stories. Babe's blood pressure tested fine as long as Sarah was around, but should a nurse Babe disliked come to check it, her pressure would go sky high, and she'd get "reported." This made her angrier and her numbers even higher. Finally her favorite nurse would arrive, and Babe would get off the reported list. This nurse seemed to understand that Babe's heart took little pauses and you had to wait a bit before deciding the reading was complete.

Babe had acquired her nickname as a toddler from her father because she would refer to herself as "the baby." The visiting nurses called her "Margaret." Nonie called her "Peg" in front of the visiting nurses but used "Babe" within the family. She really did not approve of a mature woman being nicknamed "Babe." She was "Maggie" to my mother and "Babe" to Ellen and me. Funny the number of different names a person can answer to and still be the same person.

Babe and Nonie had funds to hire Jeanette, a local woman highly recommended for her skill and compassion. She came to our home for about six hours each day, and this freed me for other responsibilities. Jeanette was great. They loved her. She did everything for them. She even cut their toenails. I would come to understand what a gift that was later on, after we lost her. Though unknown to us when she arrived, Jeanette was already dying of cancer.

Although no longer working outside the home, I cared for my grandson three days a week. He had been born a little over a year earlier. My daughter, Anita, and her husband lived in the next town, and both worked. Children have always been my favorite people. Now I had a new tummy to tickle and more little toes to kiss. The old folks loved him. Even my mother managed to laugh when the little guy climbed up her cane and she couldn't move.

"He's a nice little kid," she had said.

This made up for her awful comments when he'd been born almost five weeks early.

"When are they going to baptize that fetus?" she'd question mockingly.

Since Trevor wasn't baptized until a chubby one year old, her question had been repeated for a while. *The Mother* who had bounced light bulbs off my father's head as he'd taught my catechism had become a superstitious, rule-conscious Catholic. I suppose she feared Trevor might expire without benefit of a placement in some legalistic God's role book.

My mother, Babe, and Nonie were actually civil when they sat together during family celebrations. Babe had won family fame for her joke telling over the years, and Ellen or I would always insist she tell one of her stories. She had quite a repertoire, and how I wish we had recorded them ten years earlier, before they had to be told through loose dentures.

Those dentures! During a lunchtime munch on a turkey sandwich a bridge of false teeth loosened and trapped the meat. Babe began to choke.

"Let's stay calm," I said. "You can do this. You've dealt with that old bridge for years."

She began to laugh so I thought she'd choke again until she finally did relax and remove the tangled mess.

"Life is wasted on the young," Babe exclaimed, as she did so often.

If my mother was nearby she would always answer, "Old age is not for sissies."

Because Nonie adjusted to our life together, Babe adjusted, and we all relaxed. Ellen arrived to help as often as her life would allow. Ellen and I, our children and grandchildren, all laughed and sang with them as often as possible. We refreshed our better memories of childhood with Babe and Nonie, and our mother seemed to laugh and feel she belonged. It was a pleasant time, and we enjoyed preparing for the Christmas season.

To my surprise, it turned out to be a wonderful Christmas. I was concerned they'd be homesick, but Babe and Nonie seemed at home. Greetings and flowers came to them from their New York City friends, and they were surrounded with love and laughter.

An Indigo Bunting

Holiday decorations had hardly been returned to their basement storage shelves, when late one evening I discovered Nonie molded into her recliner. Light from a full moon slipped through a window and touched her nakedness. Sitting motionless, she appeared as a shimmering marble sculpture.

Was I in some strange museum? No, Babe was in her bed snoring as Babe had always snored. Some force seemed to have turned Nonie into stone and displaced the aunt of my lifetime. I felt frightened as if traveling alone down a dark and unfamiliar corridor.

"Aren't you cold?" I asked.

"Aren't you cold?" I repeated again.

"What are you doing here?" the statue mumbled as marble melted back to human flesh.

I guided Nonie back into bed and covered her with blankets.

Bill and I decided to set up a baby monitor so we could listen for problems during the night from our bedroom, instead of waking throughout the night and making endless journeys to Babe and

Nonie's room to discover troubles. Bill could sleep through anything unless I stirred him to help, which I kept to a minimum because he was still teaching. The newly installed technology wouldn't bother him at all. I hoped for more slumber while evaluating downstairs events from my own bed.

As I secured the device in my aunts' room, a little red light glistened. Babe wanted to know what it was, so I explained how she could now call me anytime during the night. It never dawned on Babe that I could hear her, Nonie, and everything else, even when she wasn't summoning me for help.

Their arguments during the night, once but a distant burble, now permeated our bedroom. Babe tried to convince Nonie to wear her robe. It upset Babe when she would ditch the only piece of clothing she would tolerate. Nonie now believed that even the nightgown under her robe was too harsh. As always, Nonie did her own thing. Often I lay in bed, listening to their disagreements. Occasionally, exhausted, I would turn off the monitor and hope I'd find them alive in the morning.

Thank heavens Babe and Nonie had been able to hire Jeanette! If my only release from their care had been the very few hours provided by the visiting nurses, I don't believe I would have survived what was daily intensifying as a physical and emotional drain. When morning came and Jeanette arrived I could go back to bed to snatch some lost sleep.

While ever cheerful and optimistic, Jeanette took more and more morphine for her painful shoulder. Years ago an undiagnosed squamous cell skin cancer had invaded a finger and was now taking over her body. Her work was life to her. She was determined Nonie would get better and live, as she was determined she, too, would recover and live.

Sole determination has its limits, so Jeanette's determined efforts could not slow Nonie's decline. Nonie was beginning to confuse morning and evening. She became more and more fixated upon her sister's care, and ever more frantic about producing lists, even as her handwriting became illegible.

Soon her lists stopped, and she wrote no more. She was becoming weaker and less able to walk. The jerky shakes she'd experienced in the NYC hospital were now becoming horrific.

Nonie began to believe the TV reflected dangerous invaders. She did not want to watch it any longer. She was presenting as a paranoid, jealous, nasty personality, more and more a stranger. She even became spiteful towards Babe.

"Look at her eating away over there, God love her," Nonie snapped scornfully.

As her ability to walk continued to deteriorate, she'd taunt Babe.

"Look at her dancing around, God love her. She's almost one hundred. Would you ever know?"

Her sarcastic tone hurt Babe's feelings. The same words that might have been said with Irish humor months earlier were no longer light-hearted. As always, Babe tried to soothe Nonie and make life easier for all.

I wanted to move Babe to another room to protect her and provide her with more rest. I suggested we establish the other half of the now divided living room as another bedroom. Babe would not hear of it. They were to stay together.

Babe's dictate reigned. I realized she still needed to feel like an adult with some level of control over her existence. Though she needed care, I realized she would always perceive me as the young person for whom she should make life better, as she had always done.

As Nonie's ability to walk declined, we made the mistake of giving her a folding walker. Soon we realized that learning to use any type of walker was impossible for a person forgetting how to walk. One day she attempted to stride through the thing; it folded up and she fell onto the rug in a tangled mound of flesh and metal. Bill differentiated her from it and lifted her into bed. She was a ghastly color. We could not see her breathing. She looked dead. When she opened her eyes I felt a guilt-ridden sadness she was alive. I felt sorrow for her and for myself.

Even from the distance of her apartment, my mother found Nonie's illness frightening and rarely wanted to visit inside the main house. With Jeanette on duty, I was able to maintain her schedule of shopping, lunch, and doctor visits. Her head hung down more, and her legs became weaker, but her level of overall impairment increased slowly. She gazed upon vestiges of winter's disappearance outside her glass door, and watched for signs of crocuses, daffodils and tulips. She was secure in her own space, away from the ravages of Nonie's rapid dementia.

By the end of March most of Nonie's capabilities had fled. She had forgotten how to chew and ate only blended food. Her feet crossed one over the other if she attempted to walk even while being supported. Day and night were all the same to her, and she had no clue if she had eaten ten minutes after a meal, or if she had been to the potty. She could no longer wipe her own bottom. She experienced even more frequent and more severe tremors.

So Nonie and I prepared for the ordeal of yet another visit to the doctor. I positioned her into the wheel chair we had acquired for these trips, and Bill helped move her into my car. She only weighed about 95 pounds. I imagined my chunky self as an old lady and pictured what a pain I'd be for a caregiver so desired to become very thin before I got extremely old! As we drove along I could not ignore the constant jerking of her arms and legs.

She began crying out, "I'm afraid I'll go to Hell. I'm afraid I'll go to Hell."

Nonie's screams were not the demanding, blame thrusting sort of exclamations that could come from *The Mother*. Nonie was not demanding. She was frightened. Always a person in control, she no longer had any control. Her mind had begun its descent into irrational realms of terror.

Our ride took an endless twenty minutes.

After the doctor had examined Nonie, I wheeled her into the restroom. In the bathroom she thought she saw bugs crawling all over the floor. She wanted to smash them all, and was almost falling in some vain attempt to kill them. I called for help and the doctor herself arrived.

After Nonie was soothed back into the wheelchair for the return trip, her doctor took me aside.

"It won't be long," she said.

The doctor introduced Haldol. It seemed to calm her for a few weeks before her terror returned in full force. The speed of her dementia was beyond the predictions of medicine, and help was always too little, too late.

The tremors would return. She'd make gulping sounds while trying to drink, drooled constantly, and tipped back as I maneuvered her from place to place. She become paranoid again and nasty to Babe with renewed vengeance.

Although she'd lost basic physical capabilities, she remembered other realities. She always knew who I was, who Babe was, who Bill was, who Ellen was, and where we all fit into the scheme of things.

When I questioned her about this she said, "My mind works in patches."

On a beautiful April day as the sun gleamed through the window, Nonie grabbed my hand in her paper-thin, bony one.

Desperately she demanded, "Tell me what's wrong with me."

"As you said in New York City, you are very, very ill. You are dying because your brain has some problem," I replied.

"I have holes in my head," she answered.

Then in a soft, conspiratorial voice she added, "We know the truth. The rest of them are stupid—stupid dopes. We have a secret."

For a few weeks I was the only person she wanted near her. Everyone else in the world was a stupid dope. There was no reasoning with her. This was just the way it was.

Unfortunately, we had to give Jeanette a vacation. She could not accept Nonie was dying, as she could not accept her own death. I would find her endlessly perambulating Nonie. Nonie would cross one foot over the other as Jeanette dragged her forward, straining and paining her own cancerous shoulder. We had to stalemate this pathetic chess game with death, knowing the actual and unavoidable event would be too upsetting for Jeanette.

While Jeanette rested in her own home, Ellen came frequently to fill the gap left without Jeanette's services.

Then the real nightmare began.

The constant screaming started. As during our automobile ride to the doctor's office, Nonie was frightened. She was completely terrified. Her Haldol was increased, and we thought her mind could be controlled with the medication for a while anyway, so Bill left on a scheduled two-week trip to Bahrain. I wished I could have left for the Middle East!

"Mary, Maarrrrrry," Nonie screamed.

I would hear my name endlessly. At night I'd descend the stairs and swing her onto her potty, tuck her back in bed and stumble to my room. Soon it would start again.

"Maarrry, Maaarrrrry," screeched the monitor near my bed.

Babe would get mad at her.

"Mary needs her sleep. It's the middle of the night. Mary was just here. Go back to sleep," Babe would argue.

"Maarrry, Maarrrrrry," Nonie would scream.

Down I'd go and hoist her onto the potty again. One exhausting night I felt like swinging her to Mars or Jupiter.

Then Nonie got mad at God. Apparently she had made some pact with Him that if she didn't eat anything for the entire weekend she would die by Monday. She kept asking about the days to try to keep them straight. When Monday came and she was alive she decided He had not kept His half of the bargain. After all Nonie was the frustrated businesswoman, and a bargain was a bargain. God was supposed to be a good business partner and honor His agreements, even when they were her own projections.

Tired of climbing stairs all night I made a bed out of the couch in the remaining half of the living room. I opened the door to Babe and Nonie's room located in Bill's temporary wall so I might respond quickly to the tragedy of her tormented mind.

I snuggled under a comforter and tried to sleep as I listened to Nonie rage against God.

"Look what He did to the poor Pope," she howled. "Poor Pope fell.

Look what He did to me. No bargain, no bargain."

I could not sleep. I took my pulse and it was 125. I began to get hysterical.

"I'm going to have a stroke and die, and she's still going to be here screaming at God," I told myself.

I took a deep breath. Took more deep breaths.

"Peace, Mary."

I struggled to place myself in the presence of my God. I wrangled with my soul to transcend panic and feel Love. I focused on my breathing as if about to give birth, relaxing into it as I found the rhythm of my inner being.

"Relax, breathe, and give birth to your peace. Relax, breathe and give birth to transcendence. Relax, breathe and give birth to your Love."

My pulse came down to 85. Nonie kept on screaming at God. Babe kept on telling her to go to sleep. Eventually, Nonie fell asleep.

I went to check her. With a pulse around 130, her breathing would taper off and eventually stop. Sometimes I would count to thirty. Then she would gasp and breathe. This cycle would begin again.

The visiting nurse came and catheterized Nonie, who was happy about this as it freed her from a big concern. I called Ellen. She would want to be here.

When Ellen arrived she immediately checked Nonie. Ellen was a nurse.

"Mary," she called. "Couldn't you have exaggerated for once in your life? What do you mean a little trouble breathing? I just counted to 30 before she gasped. What do you mean her urine is a little discolored? It's black, Mary. That's necrosis."

Whatever it was called, it taught the smell of death. A sweetish, sickening order permeated the room. It could not be scrubbed away, impressing itself forever into my spirit.

"You are but mortal flesh. You too will die," it taunted me.

Nonie was not to be tormented forever.

A few days after Bill returned from his two weeks in Bahrain, something happened. Suddenly Nonie became fully herself. She was her most tender, humorous and relational self. She was Nonie. She spoke to Babe about eternal life, and how they would be together again with their brother and parents. She said a beautiful good-bye to Babe, as Babe sat holding her hand. We said the *Our Father* together, Babe, Nonie, Ellen, and I. She spoke lovingly to us all. She expressed deep gratitude for her care and our home.

Our youngest son came over from the four-star restaurant where he was working as a *sommelier* to earn money for his master's degree. He came dressed in his tuxedo with the silver wine tasting cup around his neck. Nonie recognized him immediately and was so excited to greet her handsome guest. His sister rushed over. Nonie told her she loved her, what a wonderful family she thought we had, and how very grateful she was to us all.

We rejoiced with Nonie and enjoyed her prelude to heaven for about two days whenever she was awake. We exchanged peaceful farewells to our earthly relationships with her. We expressed confidence that our connections would survive the grave.

Then suddenly, without warning, that window closed. Her dementia reigned again. I knew of its return when I heard the high-pitched scream.

"Maarrrrry, Maaarry."

During the next few days, Ellen and I comforted Nonie as we could. We fed her tiny spoonfuls of sherbet, and wiped her face with a damp washcloth. Her pulse remained very high and her breathing erratic. The human body can be so fragile, and yet I wondered at its resilience even in the face of death.

Finally she began to slip into a coma. She became more rigid, and although she moaned a deep groan as a visiting nurse bathed her, she was unconscious.

It was her last bath. Pink froth began to bubble up from her lungs.

We moved Babe to another room. She accepted this, wanting only her memory of the farewell she had been able to exchange with Nonie. Babe was reassured Nonie was not suffering. She expressed satisfaction that she had done all she could for her sister, and seemed relieved to be able to shuffle away from the final scene.

Ellen and I gently wiped off the pink foam. I stepped away for a few minutes. Ellen was with her when her breathing stopped yet again, but this time never resumed. Babe's favorite nurse came to pronounce Nonie's death and to comfort Babe.

Her examination completed, Sarah, Ellen and I were standing in the kitchen looking out at the bird feeder Nonie had enjoyed so recently. With a brilliant, exquisite flash of blue, an indigo bunting landed on the feeder. Hopping to the ground it flirted its beauty in all directions. It soared up to a tree branch and danced, its iridescent hue catching the sunlight. Fluttering around but for a few moments, it disappeared. Never had it been seen before and never has it been seen since.

"Thanks, Nonie. Farewell, Nonie. Thanks."

Our daughter gave birth to another beautiful boy one week later on a radiant day in May. I had more little toes to kiss and another tummy to tickle.

One Cry

Jeanette returned, and when she wasn't caring for Babe she cradled my new grandson, gently rocking back and forth. Her daughter had announced a first pregnancy, but Jeanette seemed to know she would never live to welcome her little one. Our infant was her surrogate future. She stared into his face with the gaze of one looking ahead through the vale of imminent death.

Babe enjoyed her company, and they would often chat as Jeanette cuddled the baby. When I'd see her painful shoulder begin to sag, I'd gently confiscate him and head upstairs.

Upstairs I had another life. Soon after Babe and Nonie's arrival, we arranged our private space on the second floor. The master bedroom was turned into a family room affording comfortable couches, books, phone, and video-sound system. The remaining rooms became, respectively: our bedroom, a toy-filled children's room, and a storage area for possessions that had come with our elders. This room inspired my vow to bequeath or throw out all my stuff long before I die! To this day I still find dispossessed bits and pieces. Recently I poured the contents of a small brown envelop onto the kitchen table only to discover ancient gold teeth, kept I presume, for the gold.

Our escape zone was completely necessary for psychological survival. The baby and his two-year old brother arrived three days a week while their parent's worked, and we would ascend to this space after a "hello" to the downstairs crew. During Nonie's darkest hours their paternal grandmother had cared for them, but now we were back to the three-day routine. They brought sunshine to my tedium as I crawled around, playing on the floor.

My gardens offered another means of renewal as I savored burrowing my bare hands into the dirt while planting a new species or attacking weeds. Each perennial was a friend known by name. Moving in the warm sun and soft breeze was a pleasurable release from nervous tension. Over the years, hiking near Summerhouse in the Colorado Rockies had taught me the mental health benefits of exercise. When feeling down, get up and move. Getting up and going is always the big challenge.

On a beautiful late spring afternoon, I was weeding a flower garden situated both outside my mother's sliding glass door, and one of Babe's windows. The Belmont horse race in New York was about to begin, and I figured my dad's spirit was checking out the possible Triple Crown. Each woman came to their respective glass panel and yelled for me to come watch it with them. Being but one person I convinced Babe to invite my mother over to her television. Just in time, I convinced my mother to visit Babe's room. We all enjoyed the race and each other's company, although my mother commented she had been spooked because she believed Nonie's ghost was floating around Babe's room somewhere.

My mother looked like a ghost. Her skin color was ashen. Medical exams revealed nothing except her increasing weakness and arthritis. She still insisted on doing her own grocery shopping, but hobbling up and down the aisles with a droopy head was becoming extremely difficult.

So came the trip when she decided to drive one of those motorized carts for the handicapped. The store manager taught her how to use it and she took off. Up and down the aisles she blasted oblivious to any other human being on earth, as usual.

I could not catch her!

I really did not want to know her!

Finally, she made a grand sweep around a corner and crashed into another woman's cart. There was a big fight. The manager arrived, the very man who had taught my mother how to operate the cart minutes earlier.

"Lady," he said, "it's the same principle as when you drive a car. You must look where you are going."

"I never drove a car," retorted my defiant mother.

Following this disastrous experience, my mother gave me a list and I did her shopping.

By the fall of 1994 it was obvious that rest and relaxation would not get Babe's health back to where it had been before her effort on Nonie's behalf. We now knew she was suffering from heart failure, but she wanted no medical help. The only medicine she permitted was her four o'clock glass of wine, which she extended to two glasses. Her afternoon ritual seemed to make life worth living, and she dramatized it for all it was worth.

On one occasion after her wine time, she shuffled out to the kitchen where I was preparing dinner.

"I'm feeling a little pixilated," she stated.

I was forced to pull out the dictionary. There really was such a word.

Occasionally we tried to cut her wine with water so she would feel less "pixilated" but she always caught us.

"This wine is not very good," she would say shaking her head and grimacing.

We struggled to control the progress of her heart failure with diet but her shuffle worsened to a stumble, and she needed a walker. For a brief period she attempted to exercise by laboriously maneuvering to the front of the house and climbing the first two steps of the staircase. Soon this became impossible for her.

But she remained in charge of what she would or wouldn't do or try to do, or at least we did our best to let her think she was in charge. I never left a wine bottle in her room, but always served her cocktail hour. Should she down a bottle of wine, fall, and create more pain for herself I believed I'd be responsible because I felt I could predict the possibility. But I did not force her to exercise, play board games, or even go out to a lunch. It was a constant balancing act to protect Babe's life while leaving her personally responsible for herself.

Should I live to be very old I will have had experience with advanced age and hope to empathize with those attempting to accomplish what they believe best for me. But should I live to be very old I might forget all these lessons! A person well into the nineties needs to feel in control as much as possible, even when not able to control very much.

Babe spoke about how hard it was to be the last person from her family still alive. I reminded her that Ellen and I were family, but clearly she meant her generation. I wondered how I would feel if all my contemporaries had died, knowing parts of myself would have been lost with the death of each loved one. Every day Babe mentioned how relieved she was to have outlived Nonie. She spoke as one who had completed a mission.

I had not wept when Nonie died. The whole experience had been like a roller coaster with a sinister destination, traveling faster than my capacity for thought or emotional integration. As I grew distant from her death, the person she had been to me throughout my entire life eventually began to overshadow the nightmare of her dementia. Since this time I have spoken with many who feared their love for a significant other had been destroyed by the various factors leading to their death, but I can say with confidence that the negative feelings do not last. With time the loved one re-emerges in the full glory of their essential nature.

Nonie was beyond being frightened by the television, so once again Babe was able to enjoy this connection to the outside world. I had certain programs I watched with her while Jeanette preferred others. We could not engage Babe in any other activity. I bought books on tape, as this retired English teacher had loved literature, but she wanted nothing to do with them. Oftentimes she would simply want to sit.

"I'm meditating," she would state. "I'm almost one hundred."

It was a decree to let her be, which I obeyed. I had no clue what it would feel like to be over ninety-five. Meditation was her favorite pastime. Maybe she visited another realm wherein she frolicked with her friends and relatives.

They were all Irish, I realized one evening as I sat with her watching the News. The television blared endlessly about an African-American sports superstar on trial for the murder of his white wife. Babe watched the OJ Simpson trial and said she felt the woman's death was the expected result of her marriage to a black man. Could this be my Babe who was so devoted to her Christian faith? Perhaps she thought Jesus was Irish. Maybe she was losing oxygen to her brain from heart disease. I couldn't accept she'd expressed such a bigoted concept.

But then I knew she could, as I imagined myself back on 20th Street, my home following my dad's death. Once again I saw boats on the East River. I'd taken comfort watching them after Babe severely reprimanded me for bringing a group of young Africans to our apartment. These men were delegates to the United Nations from various countries, and I had been honored to help welcome them to the United States.

Yet I'd been horrified when they were unable to get a taxi and asked, "Why should we look for a colored cab? What color should we get?"

They had been equally confused when barbers refused to cut their kind of hair. These newly deplaned, playful African men did not understand the racism they'd encountered. I'd been ashamed as I attempted to explain the prejudice within our country.

I remembered walking into the United Nations during an African conference and turning my head to the right. This entire entrance wall was a mirror. I saw my face in the middle of all those beautiful ebony faces and didn't recognize myself. I'd felt like one of them, and

I thought my reflection was that of some ghost! I scared myself and was no longer only Irish.

Babe was certainly Irish, though her father and brother had been known as "black Irish." The family name, O'Donovan, had originated from the Irish, *O donnabhain*. It means the dark-eyed, dark-skinned ones. Babe believed they'd come to be dark due to the Spanish Armada's arrival off the Irish coast, though historians believe those guys didn't survive to populate Ireland. Wherever our dark eyes were from, it should have softened her heart against prejudice. Her own father's stoning as a presumed rabbi should have helped.

She had excused her intolerance towards my African friends on the grounds that keeping two young women safe was a rough job.

"There's no man in the house," she'd said.

I tried to accept this as an excuse after she was anything but her gracious self to the black fiancé of a close white college friend when I'd brought them home. I made excuses for her to my friend with Babe's argument that she had no man in the house to help her. Babe was all Ellen and I had as family, and it was hard to admit she wasn't perfect. It was hard to admit she'd hurt my friend and the man she loved. And now, watching the OJ trial with this ancient woman, I had to accept my home had been polluted with prejudice.

Bill unraveled some of the mystery of her attitude for me. He said it had little to do with color and everything to do with kind. After all, he had felt her prejudice against himself. He was white, but he was German. Germans were a different kind. People should stick to their own kind. If you didn't stick to your kind you deserved what you got because you couldn't expect an outsider to protect you. Certainly this is not a "one in the Spirit, one in the Lord" attitude towards humanity capable of uniting "us" and "them." We build defensive walls, and then learn the tactics necessary to maintain them, and so cut ourselves off from growth and enrichment. Yet I came to understand her capacity for prejudice better when I visited her father's town of Rosscarbery in Ireland.

As I approached this picturesque village by the sea I saw a beautiful church steeple rising above the city. It conjured up feelings of love and eternal life that were quickly dispelled when the town residents informed me that the church had been taken over by the English, the Irish forced into hiding until they were able to build their own Roman-looking church on the other side of town. The memory of English persecution was alive and well in the twenty-first century, and the townsfolk told many tales of horror. I'd always believed that if a person could be immersed in one culture besides their own, speaking the language if possible, they might begin to touch the universal family of humankind. But it may also be that a deep animosity towards one other populace may predispose a person to prejudice. Babe certainly had no use for the English. They were not her kind.

But Babe abhorred the suffering of any other humans, especially children. When the agony of the Rwanda disaster glared before us on the News, she told me to send a contribution to aid these Africans, though I'm sure it wasn't as large a contribution as it would have been for Irish children.

I'd taken over my mother's grocery shopping but she continued to look pallid and now seemed to be losing strength at a more rapid rate. I suggested she return to her doctor and made another appointment for her, but we never kept that appointment.

A few days beforehand, while I was in the kitchen preparing lunches, I thought I'd heard one barely audible cry through the closed window to her apartment. I ran next door and found her unconscious on the bedroom floor, her face a ghastly white.

I called an ambulance, and medical personnel arrived quickly and placed her on a stretcher. Then they maneuvered her out the sliding glass doors, through the garden she loved, and off to the hospital.

Ellen arrived within a few hours, and we waited to see if four blood transfusions and treatment for a bleeding ulcer would bring her around. I felt sad for the pathos and turmoil of her life but no sorrow at the thought of losing her. For a few minutes I felt the old guilt I'd felt as a child when I had wished she'd die. Yet it was clear that Ellen and I would not have been sitting in a hospital if I'd missed her cry for help. I had heard it and responded, as any honest appeal must be answered.

She survived. She also passed through the first three days of nicotine withdrawal in an unconscious state. The hospital was a smoke-free facility.

The doctors lectured that smoking and her severe ulcer were a bad combo. Her arthritis medicine was also changed, and she was told not to drink so much tea.

She was given a walker because she was much too weak and unsteady for her cane. This made her angry. She did not want to look as old as Babe or as ill as Nonie had been. The hospital staff insisted and took away her cane. They repeated often how fortunate she was not to have broken any bones. She bitched and lamented. She wanted a cigarette.

After almost twelve days in the hospital, she was released and returned home under a contract that she must accept help from the visiting nurses and home-health aides. Although she didn't want all those people in her apartment, accepting the contract freed her to leave. She was beginning to adapt to life without cigarettes, and decided to leave it that way. To her credit, she never smoked again.

My mother and Babe joined Bill, children, grandchildren, and myself for the 1994 Christmas celebration. Only a year earlier Babe, Nonie and my mother had first come together in our home, yet I felt as if that were ten years ago.

Jeanette did not celebrate with us. A couple of weeks before Christmas she had been forced to leave her work as the cancer spread rapidly from her shoulder, up her neck and towards her brain. She died two months later. When Bill and I visited the funeral parlor we prayed that our gratitude for the dedication she'd brought and the love of life she'd imparted would ring through the heavens.

Welcome Folks

My relatives were not the only elders in our immediate family. Bill's parents were ninety-two years ancient. Until ten years earlier Grandma and Grandpa had periodically driven up to visit. They would stay for less than three days.

"Fish and company stink after three days," Grandma would chirp as they departed.

During northern winter cold they had lived in Florida, then avoided its southern summer heat by returning to New Jersey. Eventually traveling became too difficult and they abandoned the seasonal change. Later they could no longer drive to Massachusetts so we all visited them. Our children loved to fish with Grandpa off the docks in Cape May.

Finally there were no more fishing expeditions as they moved near Bill's sister Jane's family in Virginia. Grandpa had realized he could no longer care for Grandma. She was becoming more and more forgetful.

"She's lost her mind," he'd announce sadly.

Also, he was trying to ignore severe intestinal problems.

They entered an assisted-living complex in Virginia Beach where they received meals in a common dining hall and had no household maintenance to fuss over. They could manage comfortably within this framework. Jane continued to assist and assess them periodically, easier for her now that they lived closer.

Grandpa finally gave away his car. It had been quite a struggle to induce him to relinquish it. What a relief! No more worry that this visually impaired, impulsively irritated, unsteady, and rather weak man would annihilate himself or another. Perhaps it would help to teach teens from the start that the engine of personal power is not to be equated with an auto engine. Perhaps it would help to prepare the young adult that as they were once too young to drive, someday, if they are fortunate, they will be too old.

Bill and I had visited Grandma and Grandpa's new residence before going to see Babe and Nonie for the last time in New York City. During that hot summer visit, Grandma had toured us through their quarters, and then we rode the elevator down to the dining room.

Upon our return from this evening meal Grandma said to me, "Come in, Mary. Let me show you where we live."

She gave me the whole tour again.

Following Babe and Nonie's arrival at our home, Bill visited his parents a number of times, but I did not go to Virginia after the summer stopover. With three very ill relatives in my care, I never traveled more than two hours from home.

Then, with the dawn of 1995, we received another disturbing phone call.

Grandma and Grandpa were in trouble.

The Folks, as we'd long called them, had been on their way to dinner when the elevator door closed on Grandma and threw her to the floor. Why any residence for the elderly did not have an elevator door that popped open on contact became a question I never felt was properly addressed. Nonetheless, addressing that issue would not have fixed Grandma. Her hip was broken, her wrist was broken, and she had lacerations on her head.

After surgery, her mind became much more confused. I wondered if anesthesia had accelerated her dementia. She was sent to a rehabilitation center for a month of physical therapy. A compliant person, she had learned to perambulate the corridors with a walker but soon became too weak for this. Bewildered, depressed, and withdrawn, she would not eat, and her once-chubby body became exceedingly thin. Discussions about tube feeding began, and Grandpa explained that her Living Will adamantly stated she wanted nothing of the sort. In her own handwriting she had added, "Let nature take its course."

Grandpa felt she was going to die. The rehab center felt she was going to die if she was not tube fed. This facility could not do anything more for her, and Grandpa could no longer care for her in the assisted living residence. She did not walk, she was incontinent, and she would never be able to go down for meals.

Bill's sister Jane could not take them into her home. Bill's oldest sister, Rachel, lived in Georgia. She could not do this either. Both sisters and their husbands lived busy lives that included extensive traveling. Throughout the month of this January, Bill, his sisters and Grandpa discussed Grandma's prognosis and worked on a follow-up plan.

We suggested to Grandpa that they move in with us. This time it was my idea to open our home to elderly relatives. I figured we were already so tied up, what difference would two more make? There was that empty half of the large original living room on the other side of Bill's temporary wall. It might as well be another bedroom. We couldn't use it. Our living room was now upstairs, and entertaining quests was certainly impossible these days. We went out to dinner with friends, or visited their homes when others could fill in for us.

Grandpa decided that living in his son's home would solve his problems.

Bill's two sisters, Jane and Rachel, were not happy. They are five and seven years older than Bill, and I don't know that they had ever rejoiced over his birth. Relationship had long been a source of stress.

The family had been through economically difficult years before Bill's arrival at the end of the Depression. Then a son had been born who seemed to be given all available goodies. As teens Jane and Rachel were required to peddle flowers to local florists. Grandpa grew them with the hope the sales would be a source of funds for Bill's college education. When the sisters were of college age, Jane and Rachel had been loaned money to go to secretarial school and had been required to pay it back. As girls, they were not recognized for their talents. Baby brother, "Brother Bill," appeared to get it all, and their slave labor besides. And now the old parents wanted to live with "Brother Bill."

Rachel and Jane wanted Grandma and Grandpa placed in a nursing home. Both had married into considerable wealth, so Grandpa's inheritance meant little to them. They said they didn't care if he spent it on housing and nursing care. Yet Grandpa's inheritance meant everything to him. He had saved all through his senior years to be able to leave a little money to his "heirs" as he called them, his children and grandchildren. He was obsessed with keeping count of his assets and to whom they'd be distributed. His identity and personal esteem seemed to rest with this. Perhaps it made up for having lost his farm during the Depression.

Paul, our youngest son, and Grandpa often exchanged letters wherein Grandpa would remind him, "A penny saved equals a penny earned."

Grandpa packed some pictures and a few clothes into a suitcase, those few items he and Grandma had not already given away, and prepared to fly north. Jane settled them on the plane despite her aggravation.

As Grandpa saw it, they were arriving to die. Grandpa's plan was that Grandma would die and then he would expire a few days later. He had recently been diagnosed with colon cancer.

Bill and Paul met them at Boston's Logan Airport with our collapsible family wheelchair.

Our son never forgot this cold, gray New England winter day. On the ride into Boston he pictured his warm and friendly Grandpa and his forgetful but perky Grandma. He had not seen them in a few years due to his work and school schedules. When he and Bill arrived at the Continental Airlines terminal, they greeted four Continental staff caring for two old people in two wheelchairs. Grandpa was silent and ghostly white. Grandma appeared to have died during the trip. She was rigid and unresponsive, her face expressionless, and her color also ghastly. Somehow they loaded the Folks into our car. The trip home was made in total silence.

Arriving home, Bill wheeled Grandma up the planks he had put in place for that purpose and traversed the few steps through the entryway.

Once again the apparition of a near corpse crossed before my mother's eyes as she came out to meet my in-laws for the first time.

"You're crazy," she said quietly to me, then turned her walker back towards her door.

I thought she might have a point.

We changed Grandma's disposable pants and placed her in Nonie's unneeded recliner, tucking a blanket around her. Pale, very thin, her hands knotted and her body coiled in a fetal position, she certainly did not appear long for our world.

I held her rigid, cold, coiled hand in mine and tried to open it a little, but many of the bones were fused. She had not moved certain fingers for too long.

"Hi, Grandma." I said. "I'm Mary. I married your son, Bill. I'm the Mary of 'Mary and Bill.' You are now in our home and we are going to take care of you."

"Mary of 'Mary and Bill,'" said a little voice. "Well, well thank you for your hospitality."

She squeezed my hand lightly before her mind floated away. She was almost unconscious.

Grandpa had made it up the planks on his own. He had walked plenty of them as a carpenter, and somehow he managed to get his imbalances to balance out. He looked around his new home and was satisfied. He seemed to settle down and flush color into his face.

He was introduced to Babe. They were both sociable sorts and almost immediately seemed to enjoy talking. That night they had dinner together and exchanged stories at our kitchen table.

Then a potential problem became evident. Grandpa had learned where to find the bathroom and made use of it just as Babe was heading for the facility.

"There's a man in the bathroom," said Babe. "I guess I'll have to wait."

A disgruntled Babe shuffled back to the kitchen table to sit in line.

Our medical doctor evaluated Grandma through reports from the visiting nurses. Although she would want to examine her eventually, she wanted to see Grandpa immediately. She wanted to go over his options.

She clipped up his x-rays and discussed his records. In her expert opinion he should have surgery to prevent a possible bowel obstruction. She felt this was not an unusual life-prolonging procedure but a comfort measure. A very tall, sensitive woman, this doctor sat next to Grandpa and hugged him. Warmly she told him all the ways she would prefer to die rather than dying of a bowel obstruction.

He would not listen to her. No doctor was going to cut him open. Forget it. There was no further reasoning with him, and the discussion was over. He told the doctor his plan. His wife was going to die soon, and then he was going to die a few days later.

She enrolled him in the Hospice Program with our already visiting nurses and prescribed a huge bottle of morphine to be kept on hand. A gentle person, this doctor cringed at the thought of Grandpa's possible suffering.

We placed the large bottle of morphine on a top shelf in our kitchen. The same shelf held Grandma's only pill and Babe's blood pressure medication. As this new bottle of blue liquid shimmered above, it seemed an ominous admonition that we might have difficult days ahead.

Hello Again, Will

As a lifetime hobby I'd enjoyed reading medical literature, probably to keep in touch with my youthful aspiration. Therefore, I'd learned that the elderly are sometimes poisoned by digitalis as they become sensitive to their dose. Weight loss can enhance the maladjustment.

I soon discovered the medication resting on my shelf for Grandma was actually digitalis with a fancy name. She'd been given it fifteen years earlier after she had passed out once. Never had she undergone any tests on her heart nor had there been any indication of heart trouble. Her dose had never been adjusted. I guess taking this pill had become some kind of habit any new doctor had simply continued. Presently, her blood pressure was so low and her pulse so slow, she barely breathed. Curled into an almost fetal position, she was only semi-conscious.

Aware she was dying, as were the nurses, I saw no reason to feed her possible poison. I threw her tablets in the garbage.

Thereafter, day-by-day, Grandma became a bit livelier.

"Where am I?" she asked.

"This is your son Bill's house. I am Mary of 'Mary and Bill.' We are taking care of you here in our home."
"That is so kind of you. Where do you live?"
"In Massachusetts. You are in Massachusetts."
"It's cold there."
"Yes, but we keep you nice and warm."
"That's very kind of you."

She began to eat and drink more. She held onto her walker and tried to get up. We steadied her and she took a few steps. We put a portable potty in her room, and she began to use it instead of her pants.

Sitting in her lounge chair she looked over at the twin bed pressed against her own. Grandpa was lying in his bed snoozing.
"Who's that man over there?" asked Grandma.
"That's your Will," I answered.
"My Will?"
"That's right."
"Let me go tickle him and find out."

With that Grandma lifted herself from her recliner, grabbed onto her bed and inched herself towards Grandpa. Yanking off his blankets she began to tickle his feet.
"Hey," he yelled. "What are you doing?"

So, Grandma's doctor praised me and officially diagnosed digitalis poisoning. Should I have felt happy about this? I wasn't sure. She still had advanced Alzheimer's disease, and I had certainly ruined Grandpa's plans!

One evening, an exhausted Grandpa passed us on his way back to bed after a bathroom trip. Grandma was at the kitchen table talking to Bill, and eating yet again.

Grandpa looked over at her and grouched, "It's time for bed and she's partying away."

He was not a happy man.

Soon Grandma could navigate herself around the house.

Although she remained thin, she was an exceedingly strong person, and she moved very fast. One day we found her in the bathroom after she'd eaten most of a bar of soap. Her teeth marks were embedded into what was left. She did not need extra fruit and vegetables that day.

She began talking, not to anyone in particular, just prattling. She had always been a very quiet person, and now the chatter seemed endless.

Her jabber aggravated Grandpa. His hearing loss prevented him from understanding what she was saying and he didn't understand that she really wasn't speaking to him. He'd holler for silence.

Grandma babbled even more during the night. This really annoyed Grandpa. After they held hands reciting good night prayers, it was supposed to be quiet time. Such had been their routine for over half a century. No more. Evening announced the hours of Grandma's greatest agitation. Often she would begin this lively period by pulling the covers off Grandpa's bed while giggling like a little girl.

Confused and angered, he would yell, "What do you think you're doing?"

Bill and I would fall asleep with his frustrations filling the night air around us through our well-used baby monitor. Babe slept soundly through it all despite sound permeating the dividing wall between herself and the Folks. She did not feel responsible for them, as she had for Nonie, so she was able to tune them out, as a mother can tune out a child not her own. We would hear her snoring in the background.

One night Bill and I desired to enjoy the tension release of good sex, perfected over many years. With my mother-in-law chattering away in our bedroom I'd found this outlet impossible. I turned off the monitor.

At some point during the night I awoke and heard the silence. No chatter. No snoring. I had forgotten to turn the machine back on so I flipped the switch. There was still complete silence.

Down the stairs I went. Grandma was not in her bed. I could not find her anywhere. I started to panic, but the doors leading outside were all barricaded with the children's plastic riding horses. Grandma always glared at those horses as if they were real. She dared not disturb them.

Where was she?

I went into Babe's room to see if my old aunt was all right. The nightlight illuminated Babe's form meditating in her recliner.

"Why aren't you sleeping?" I asked her.

"How can I?" she replied.

I looked towards her bed and there was Grandma sound asleep. Her walker was next to the bed and over it was draped the Depends diaper she wore at night.

"This happened to me when I was in the hospital for gallbladder surgery," sighed Babe. "A woman always came to sleep with me at night. Why do they want to sleep with me? They have their own beds."

"Sorry Babe," I said as I remedied the situation as fast as possible. Poor Babe, who didn't even like to be touched!

Obviously I needed to make up sleep during the day. Life was becoming much more hectic now that Grandma was living.

Babe and Grandpa agreed to join financial forces, and we hired another person to help.

We found Helen, a young mother in her early twenties, with lots of tenderness and enthusiasm. She lacked Jeanette's experience, and would not be able to cut toenails, yet her positive energy made my life much easier, and I could rest.

I couldn't cut toenails. I don't know why, but even attempting the task made me nauseous. When I think of all I did do; of the pink foam, of all the bottoms I'd wiped, of the diapers and potties, and sick stomachs, it's hard to understand. I don't know why I couldn't do toenails. It wasn't because I was afraid I'd cut off their toes.

So without Jeanette we had to find a podiatrist who would do home visits. We found one, and also an eye doctor who would check glaucoma. It was not easy, but I guess we had enough feet and pairs of eyes to make it worthwhile.

We also found a hairdresser to come. Babe would allow the professional to comb her hair, so occasionally we managed to spruce her up.

Helen was warm, efficient, and optimistic in her attention to the elders. We extended her hours to help a little with my mother. This was risky because my mother was difficult even for the cleaning service, but Helen's cheerful presence dominated.

It was fun having a younger person around. I had a chance to teach a new generation while putting one to rest. Helen accepted cooking lessons, and one day she asked me to inspect a roasting pan. Placing it before me she wanted to know if everything was satisfactory before she cooked the chicken. The chicken? That's what it was? I stared at the thing for a minute until I realized the bird had been placed in the pan upside down and rested uncomfortably on its breast. I turned it over and found the paper-wrapped giblets still lodged within the body cavity. It was good to be reminded how easily we can take too much for granted.

As Babe and Grandpa sat together and ate Helen's dinners, they told each other the same stories every evening with as much enthusiasm as they had the night before.

One evening, when back in her room, Babe pulled me aside and whispered, "You know Mary, I know every one of his stories. I even know every single comma and period."

Amazing how that proverbial speck is so much harder to see in one's own eye!

Grandma had no concern for the speck in her eye or anyone else's. She had simple, practical concerns.

Dozing in her recliner she awoke again one day to find a man sleeping in her room.

"There's a man in that bed," she said to no one in particular.

"Yes Grandma, that's your Will."

"My Will? I must poke him and see."

"Maybe he needs to sleep."

"Who are you?"

"I'm Mary of 'Mary and Bill.' I married your son Bill. I live here. You are in our house, and we are taking care of you."

"Thank you so much. That is so kind of you. And that's my Will?"

"Yes, Grandma. That's your Will."

A Final Toast

Soon after he was settled in our home Grandpa wanted to discuss the reality of dying with his daughter, Jane. He wanted to talk about how important he thought it was to accept death as part of life. Jane didn't want to think about it, and told her father she had no intention of dwelling on the subject.

"You should think about it," he had said.

And since he had so commanded, she resisted. The two of them incessantly locked heads in oppositional feuds.

When the warm spring sunshine did not tempt Grandpa outside, Jane began to accept his frailty. It was not like Grandpa to resist the outdoors on a beautiful day. He had worked in the open air all his life, and after he retired had helped out as mate on a fishing boat.

A large picture of himself had appeared in The Philadelphia Sunday Bulletin on July 20, 1969. The headline for the article read: *Philosophical Mate on Boat Helps Deep-Sea Anglers Keep Their Cool*, and went on to say:

At an age when most retired men are inclined to relax, William Moeller, 68, has an assignment that has been known to tax the stamina and skills of a much younger man.

Moeller has taken on the post of mate aboard the Ogle II, a deep-sea party fishing boat operating out of Cape May in the Atlantic Ocean and Delaware Bay.

Ask the affable wind-and-sun-tanned man why he does it, and he takes his corn cob pipe out of his mouth and declares, "I like to fish; that's why."

Now he was an indoor man, developing more serious symptoms of his progressing cancer. His skin had become very thin and exhibited a torturous itchy rash from the toxins. This condition required two salves twice a day. Should he scratch his legs, the resulting gouges created more problems. His bowels were difficult to control, so we gave him a bedside potty like Grandma's. Babe also had hers now, making potty emptying a constant chore. Grandpa often used Grandma's when he believed no one was watching so that the pink urine he produced could be blamed on her. Despite poor vision he could see enough to realize it was the wrong color.

One Saturday he hurriedly entered the regular bathroom and closed the door. He stayed a long time, and when I heard rattling and banging I went to discover his problem. The poor old man was trying to clean up excrement plastered everywhere. He had not reached the toilet. His efforts were making matters far worse, and the bathroom floor, the lavatory cabinet, and the walls were patterned with red-brown handprints. The odor was overwhelming despite the open window, and Grandpa needed a shower. I called out for Bill. Suddenly, this was clearly his father!

Bill may have been busy elsewhere on many occasions when I could have used his help during our life together, but his presence this day made up for everything. He came promptly and took over, bathing his large, strong dad, and polishing the room.

The smell of Lysol permeated the air. I came to detest that scent. I used this cleaning fluid many times a day, as it claimed to eliminate germs. Even today, a whiff of the stuff can resurrect putrid memories. Should I need to eliminate germs in the future I'd hope to find something else.

The supervising nurse recommended that Grandpa be granted more services so subsequently more health aides and volunteers came to our home. When totaling the number of professionals arriving for each elderly person, alongside family members, many persons drove up to the house. One early morning, while Bill was outside rebuilding a slight bump across our dirt driveway to divert water during storms, a regular visiting nurse stopped and asked him if he was installing a speed bump.

Personal privacy was a concept without meaning. Bill and I had to leave home to be alone, and occasionally spent a night in a local hotel while our children took over. One restful night away could feel like a week's vacation!

Arriving home following one of these brief overnights donated by our son Paul, I discovered our old mellow, white cat was no longer there.

"He's at the Vet's," Paul explained. "He didn't look too good, so I took him over. They wanted to keep him for an evaluation."

Picturing a cash register compiling dollars by the second, I rushed over. I found Chico strapped down on an examination table with an IV tube in his front leg. I was told he was dehydrated from diabetes and was then presented with a few expensive options.

I thought of our elderly dying peacefully without tubes and then looked at Chico. I promised the Vet I'd give him lots of fluids and keep him comfortable until he slipped into a coma. They unhooked my cat, I paid the bill, and we waved farewell. Chico lived over a year, caught dozens of mice, and drank lots of water.

And I did thank Paul for caring diligently for all the living creatures in our home while we rested!

During the normal run of the week, day and night blended together. Service providers slept in their own homes at nighttime while we alone were responsible. Bill, our baby monitor, and I worked together. Slumber was a luxury for me.

Grandma continued to prattle endlessly. Once she talked nonstop for eighteen hours, right through the night. Her favorite topic became a relationship to some lover. He seemed to have nothing in common with Grandpa, at least as we ever knew of him. Grandma's lover seemed to be an idealized man. Fantastically handsome, he was so gentle, romantic, intelligent, sensitive, and charming. Always tenderly attentive, he would swoop her away to many exciting places. They would laugh together and tune out the whole world.

Many persons become silent with Alzheimer's disease, but not Grandma. She had always been a very intelligent woman with great language skills and she kept her enduring verbal strength. But her endless talk was not connected to anything we understood, had experienced, or could follow logically, although she was not talking to anyone in particular anyway.

Late into a night, near the end of May 1995, with Grandma chattering away in the background, I heard Babe struggling to cough. I went down to her room and asked how she was doing.

"If I'd known you'd get out of bed and come downstairs just because I coughed I'd have lain here and choked," she exclaimed.

As I fetched Babe a drink and adjusted her pillow, I could clearly hear Grandma's continuing singsong story. Suddenly Grandpa had heard enough of the never-ending saga.

"For God's sake will you wake up and go to sleep," he shouted at his wife, whose story telling continued without missing a beat.

I examined Babe the next morning as I squeezed her eye drops for glaucoma. She was pale and her lips slightly blue. She had little strength to get to the bathroom and used her bedside potty, which she detested.

"You shouldn't be emptying that," she said. "I should be in a nursing home."

"You are in a nursing home," I said, after thanking her for changing my diapers in ages past.

She chuckled, and every day we repeated the joke.

"I should be in a nursing home."
"You are in a nursing home."

On a Friday early in June, with the doctor unavailable, Babe's favorite nurse came to see her. Ellen was visiting, and Sarah told us Babe had fluid in her lungs. Then this nurse who had always loved to stay and chat with us, turned towards the door and took off. She loved Babe, and she knew Babe wished no heroic attempts to save her failing heart. I can only believe Babe's fateful rattles upset Sarah.

This was not the first or the last time I was exposed to and affected by the emotions of providers who came to our home. Many were anxious near the dying. Some who had lost relatives recently, as this nurse had just lost a beloved grandmother, would become overwhelmed with unresolved personal feelings. Others had no familiarity with or understanding of hospice, believing sick and dying people belonged in the hospital. This was particularly noticeable because the providers originated both from the hospice program where they had been trained to console those coping with the end of earthly life, and the regular visiting nurse program staff. Some non-hospice providers, critical of hospice philosophy, struggled to honor that within our home these elders were to be gifted the personal and natural death experience they had specifically requested in writing. Others needed consolation themselves as they grieved their individual losses. Sarah had not stayed long enough for consolation.

Fortunately, this same Friday morning, the supervising hospice nurse arrived to visit Grandpa. We asked her to check Babe. She examined her, and then telephoned the doctor on call. They agreed we should use Grandpa's unopened bottle of morphine should she begin to suffer. It would be impossible to acquire any over the weekend in our area because a morphine order cannot be phoned to a pharmacist. When the heart is failing, fluid collects throughout the body and fills the lungs, just as fluid fills the lungs of the drowning. We did not want such discomfort for Babe. She was, thereupon, officially enrolled into the hospice program.

To choose a tubeless, natural death is not to choose pain.

We rented a hospital bed so we could raise her head to make her breathing a bit easier, and it arrived within a few hours.

As the medical supply company set up the new bed Babe said to me, "Mary, why are you bothering with this? I'll only need it for a few days."

She had never wanted to cause any commotion. She continuously tried to make life easier for others.

Ellen phoned her family and explained her visit had turned into a time of sorrow, and that she would remain with Babe.

The next evening, Saturday evening, we poured three glasses of wine. Ellen and I sat in chairs on either side of Babe's recliner. We held up our glasses with hers and toasted her journey to eternal life. We toasted a long distance hello to our father and to Nonie. We thanked her for the gift she was to our lives. We laughed and prayed through a soulful farewell to this mother-aunt who was, as she liked to note, "almost one hundred."

I left home afterwards to take my grandsons to a local carnival as I had promised. The flashing lights, cheap food and superficial thrills conflicted with my inner grief and increased my profound loneliness. It would be years before I could enjoy a grandson enjoying a carnival.

Ellen remained with Babe. She asked her to keep in touch from heaven, somehow, and let her know anything she could about life on the other side. Babe asked if she'd really want to know should she learn exotic information. They bantered about some "what ifs" that started Babe laughing.

"What if St. Patrick was Jewish? What if the Blessed Virgin wasn't a virgin after all? What if there were really two Gods?"

Babe almost died laughing. Her lungs were too full of fluid to sustain hilarity. The laughter turned into gasping, bubble-filled coughs. When I returned from the carnival, Ellen was shaking. Babe's near death from mirth had been terrifying.

On Sunday morning Babe watched Mass on television from her elevated bed as she sipped her precious black coffee. She was peaceful, although her breathing rattled and her lips were blue. As the day progressed she slept much of the time, and was not fully conscious.

She rallied at one point as Ellen and I stood on either side of her bed.

"What do you see, Babe?" Ellen asked.

"There are two of them," said Babe.

"Now don't start that again," retorted Ellen.

"You never cry, Mary," Babe said as we remained beside her.

I told her I do cry, but generally not in front of people. As I said this I felt a sense of failure. I knew I really had never cried very much even when alone. I wondered if I were too cut off from feeling. Perhaps I lived too much within my mind. I decided I needed more connection to my emotions and vowed not to monitor what I should and shouldn't feel. But even this inner discussion with myself was itself very intellectual. I had not cried when my father died after his three-year ordeal with cancer. The dean of my college, who had become my friend, commented on this and had asked if I'd loved him. That question had hurt and confused me. I had not cried when Nonie died. When had I really cried? Could I weep? I did not know! Babe's final admonition crept deep into my soul.

Throughout my childhood I cannot remember a single discussion about personal feelings of sadness or loss. All sorrows, no matter how traumatic, were to be offered up to God for whatever use He might have had for them. Sometimes a tragedy might be described as "for the best." When all else failed, "Christ suffered and died a violent death for us all, so what should we have to complain about?" My gentle pediatrician had not addressed my tears when I wept over my mother's mental disability. While he was dying, my father opened his oil painting sets and used art to project his identification with the suffering and death of Christ. Grief on an intimate personal level was either a void or bathed in religious symbolism. Therefore, I had always identified my own grief with the suffering of Christ rather than as a means of achieving emotional integration. This maintained a whitewash over my inner feelings, keeping them hidden even from myself.

Jane was in town to visit her father during the weekend that Babe entered hospice. She and her dad sat at the kitchen table while Ellen and I attended to Babe. Loudly, they challenged each other in their usual tug of war, and discussed the stock market. Ellen and I motioned to Jane, begging for more quiet. She came into Babe's room and looked into the hospital bed.

"What's the matter with her?" she asked.

"She's dying," I said.

"Really? Oh," replied Jane, who then left and continued her conversation with a little less gusto.

Early Monday morning Grandpa came to Babe's room. He used a walker to help his balance. It had been difficult to convince him to use one, until the day he balanced himself by bouncing off the walls, knocking pictures down in the process. Now he stood leaning on the walker and staring at Babe. It had been months since they had been able to laugh over their dinners together and tell their stories, yet he smiled sweetly.

"She's peaceful," he stated. "Dying is not so bad. Nothing to it."

He turned and left the room with a thud-slide, thud-slide, apparently comforted by this revelation.

Ellen and I decided our mother might benefit from offering a brief good-bye to Babe. She agreed to this, and we assisted her. As her slumped form sat beside the bed, she appeared again as the pathetic child who had been escorted by hospital attendants to our father's funeral. The corners of her mouth turned way down and her eyes oozed a confused aversion. She simply could not cope. She said a prayer for the "Maggie" she would miss. Babe had always been kind to her.

The hospice nurse tried to catheterize Babe, who was semi-conscious. We gave her extra medication so she would not be traumatized by this invasion of her body. She had become quite swollen with fluid from her heart failure, and this made the process very difficult. The visiting nurse could not accomplish the task, and my sister had to pull out her nursing skills to complete the job as quickly as possible. She desired to save Babe any more embarrassment or discomfort. This was traumatic for Ellen, although Babe became so serene we imagined she was offering the experience to heaven! Finally Babe was relieved and made comfortable, and a home-health aide sponged her gently.

The priest and nun who ran our parish church came and administered the last rites, expressing their warmth and respect for Babe. The priest, noticing her blue face and lips, recommended some times for the funeral. Roberta, blessed with more interpersonal skills, told him to wait until after her death to discuss the arrangements.

She died the next evening. She had begun the familiar, stop and go, Cheyne-Stokes breathing, and we counted to twenty or thirty before her next breath.

Then there simply wasn't a next breath. I really, really did cry. Ellen and I, on either side of her bed, had a good cry together.

I had made the preliminary arrangements with a funeral director for both Babe and Nonies' funerals a few months before Nonie died. At the time it had felt awfully weird to plan these events with an undertaker while loved ones were alive at home. I loathed the process despite the pleasant, calming manner of the funeral director.

Yet as the nurse was on her way to pronounce Babe's death, I was thankful I would be able to call the mortician without any need to think or plan. In the future this required task would again be simple because Grandpa had made the arrangements for his own funeral and for Grandma's. They were each to have a simple service at the funeral home, and then be cremated.

He with the calming manner, and an assistant, arrived to claim Babe's empty shell. As they placed her well-used form into a heavy, black plastic body bag, her hand flopped lifelessly, the hand that had rubbed our heads for so many years. I felt the flopping of that hand as if it were my own. I sensed the reality of my own death as if viewing my own discarded peel. For a moment I was in the black plastic bag and could no longer reach out to touch. I had loved Babe, and now a part of myself had died. To preserve myself I would preserve her within my memory, while trusting a God Who loves us all and might miss us, to preserve her in a realm beyond imagination.

Her funeral Mass helped to soothe my sorrow. Our priest asked me to speak, and I did so with my hand on her casket. I was able to acknowledge something of what she had taught throughout my life.

"Don't take yourself too seriously. Life is too short. Take the step back. Look for the humor you can always find if you can see your pain from some distance. You're never the only one in the world having a bad day, and you might not want to trade yours in for another's! Sorrow will end. Time heals, and the sun will be out tomorrow or the next day. Laugh together, and together give a toast to Life."

I removed my hand from the casket.

"Please God," I prayed silently, "may she be my special guardian angel."

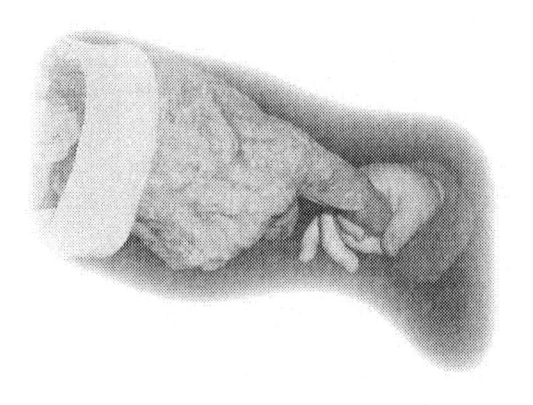

Lucking Out

Upon Babe's death, Ellen and I arranged for a celebration to honor her life. Babe had loved parties, so we planned a good one and booked a function room at a local hotel. My home was unsuitable for such an event, with living rooms now bedrooms for the dying. The entire family gathered, including our oldest son, Peter, and his daughters, from Indiana. Everyone reserved rooms in the hotel and renewed their connections. Local friends, nurses, and home-health aides arrived and joined the fun. Bill and I transported my mother and then placed her in a wheelchair she had accepted for that day only. When she tired early in the evening, Steven and his spouse generously returned her to her apartment so we could remain with our family.

I imagined my new guardian angel smiling and enjoying many good laughs as we exchanged Babe stories. Perhaps she even snuck a few sips of the best wine.

On the morning of Peter's planned return to Indiana, he sat at the breakfast table with Grandpa and his eldest child. Grandpa reached into his pocket and handed her an envelope. He was deeply moved as he presented a substantial savings bond to this oldest great-granddaughter. Always fair, he had a stack of bonds of equal amounts for each of his eleven great grandchildren. He fought back tears, as he was able to hand it to one old enough to understand, and receive her hug of thanks. I felt sad believing he would never hug this child again. I almost wept, imaging a day when I would give my own last hug to this first grandchild.

As days went by, Grandpa's fingers moved more and more slowly over the metal keys of his ancient typewriter. He typed endlessly, defining and analyzing the value of his assets. He only cared that they might benefit his "heirs." To have these "heirs" seemed to validate his life of hard labors and many difficult times. He became irritable as his fingers became weaker and more uncoordinated. When he could no longer type, he became even more irascible.

While Bill always shared our responsibilities, he had to carry on at the University, and so there were long periods each week when I had no chance for relief except when we could arrange for help. I would not have been able to survive the demands of caring for even one of our dying if our families had not been able to afford to hire Jeanette, then Helen, and now Hannah. Helen, having earned official status as a home-health aide, had found a full-time job that provided her with health insurance benefits. Hannah was a gentle mother of three, and certified aide whose husband carried their insurance.

These competent persons had given me, and now in the person of Hannah gave me, the chance to get some distance from unending, grueling demands. The aides supplied by Medicare, and the volunteers from the hospice program, afforded an hour or so of break here and there, which was so important. However, I needed more time than that to unwind and enjoy caring for my grandchildren, balance the checkbook, do the shopping, take a nap after a bad night, work in my gardens, or relax and listen to music. After a good break with Hannah on duty, I could return to active caring with renewed vigor.

I am sure many could be spared the communal isolation and expense of nursing home placement if families received more support to keep sick and dying relatives at home. The public health system could save money if it would supply sufficient assistance towards that purpose. Residency at a nursing home is becoming more and more costly, rapidly depleting such family funds as Grandpa wanted to leave his heirs. And once all those funds have vanished and families have lost what they had worked years to obtain for grandchildren, government must continue to fund treatment unless we want to become a nation tossing the dying onto the street. It makes sense to support families who want to keep relatives at home by providing them with adequate relief because it is an impossible task without adequate relief. A few consecutive hours away are essential to a caregiver's health. Fortunately, we were able to hire private assistance, but many families cannot afford to become employers.

Predictably at noon each day, an irritable Grandpa would thump his walker into the kitchen. He would sit down and then shake the metal bars beside him if his peanut butter and jelly sandwich was not there waiting for him. Should I continue to be occupied, the pounding walker became a loud, frustrated demand. He'd been served this sandwich or had it packed for him almost every day of his adult life. Should his angry noise mount at the absence of his sandwich and cup of coffee, I'd fight off irate feelings. I reminded myself he was a sick, ninety-four-year-old man from a different era, and this was not a time to update him.

It was also hard for me to bump into the rigid, angry, dogmatic side of Grandpa because until that time I had never experienced him as anything but a warm, accepting, and affectionate person. Grandma had always impressed me as the physically distant one. Whenever I had watched her with my infants, I had been amazed at how far out from her body she'd hold them. Her hands were never soft and gentle. Even as advancing age and the dulling effect of Alzheimer's were taking their toll on all aspects of her vitality, her hands still grabbed my arm with a steel-hard grip. As long as I'd known her, she had spoken often about her lack of maternal feelings and skills, and her notion that if she hadn't been influenced by "biology," she would have been better off remaining the business woman she had been and had enjoyed being. She had described Grandpa to me as the teddy bear. He was the hugger. He provided warmth. I had believed her, because this was how I had experienced him.

However, he did not have an open mind. She did. She was always a free spirit interested in new ideas and always searching to understand more. So, the aloof one welcomed your unconventional thoughts, and the warm one turned suddenly rigid and ice cold if you crossed some invisible line you didn't know existed.

I hadn't known this until I'd witnessed his interactions with Jane, and until I, the woman, the housefrau, didn't have lunch on the table at noon. It was a distressing shock to discover that the back of the teddy bear was of different cloth than the front.

As his disease advanced, he became more rigid, as Grandma was becoming freer, and as Babe had become more serene. Some basic personality seems to take over in the end as our pretenses begin to fail us along with our vitality. After having observed this several times, I would advise against holding out for a great deathbed conversion. We sure are who we are in the end. Better that we dump our facades, open up and soften our inner selves as soon as possible!

Yet illness can take its toll on personality. During times I felt irritated at Grandpa's grumpiness and dogmatism, I told myself to dig up compassion. I could not know what effect his cancer was having on his disposition. I didn't know what parts of his body were being ravaged. What caused the red urine? Were his brain and liver involved? He was not interested in knowing anything about it, but we needed to remember destructive things were happening to him. He was becoming weaker and more confused whether from cancer or toxins from cancer.

I went downstairs late one night to calm Grandpa when I heard him becoming agitated. I chose not to awaken Bill and ask for help because he had an appointment the following day. Grandpa was out of bed. He said he was crawling through a long tunnel. He wanted to get through it to something he saw at the other end. I tried to maneuver him back to bed but became trapped between this powerful man's attempt to get somewhere, and the wall. Pinned there, I called out for Bill, who finally heard me over the monitor. He guided his dad back to bed and gave me a lecture. I was not to manage him alone. Well, I'd learned I couldn't do that. Even when dying, he was stronger than I.

A few nights later we heard Grandpa crashing around the house and discovered him searching for and finding the whiskey. This was not like him. He'd always enjoyed one small nightcap before retiring, so a 2 A.M. quest for the bottle was out of character.

The doctor decided he was in pain, would not admit to it, and was trying to medicate himself. She started him on the blue liquid morphine. Babe had not used much of it.

Grandma added to his burdens. She did not prattle quite as much anymore, but she had started something new. She spoke only German. A German woman had been assigned to them as their home-health aide. She addressed Grandma as "Frau Moeller," and spoke to her in German. After this, Grandma spoke only German. Grandpa became furious at this. He groused that she had only learned German in high school while it was his primary language.

"Why is she speaking it now? She would never speak to my mother in German when I wanted her to. Why now?"

Of course, we explained her brain was not functioning rationally, but then neither was his. We attempted to define her disease for him, but his own disease hampered comprehension. They had been a couple for over sixty years, and yet we were trying to tell them about each other.

Around midnight on a rainy night, we heard Grandpa yelling at Grandma over our monitor. He sounded exceedingly distraught. Bill flew to his parent's room and found his father standing beside his wife's bed with a pillow lifted high over his head. Was he going to smack or smother her? We will never know, but Bill halted him and returned him to bed.

We decided keeping Grandma and Grandpa together in the same room was a nonsensical sentimentality benefitting neither of them. He seemed upset by anything she did, and she didn't know who he was. What was the point?

We moved Grandma's twin bed and chair into Babe's old room. Speaking English again, she asked if her potty was located in a different place than it had been, but never wondered where Grandpa had gone. Grandpa didn't say much about Grandma's disappearance. He failed rapidly and was becoming semi-conscious. He slept most of the time and was confused and upset when awake. He had not moved his bowels in a few days, and we feared an obstruction might have caught up with him. We feared an episode of "Moeller Luck."

Through many difficulties and bad turns over the years, Grandma had come to classify life in the family as continuously subject to "Moeller Luck." This verbalized her conviction that the worst thing possible was always bound to happen.

The hospice nurse arrived frequently to visit Grandpa. One afternoon she felt him struggling with emotions, though he was almost comatose, and told him he had nothing to worry about. She declared he could leave this world because Bill and I would take good care of his wife, "Ceil." This seemed to have an immediate and extremely soothing affect upon Grandpa. Although not able to speak, he released a deep sigh.

Shortly after the nurse had left, Hannah and I were standing on either side of Grandpa's bed, attempting to make him comfortable. Then we noticed he was slipping out of consciousness. Hannah wiped Grandpa's brow with a damp cloth, and then we tried to arrange his long legs so they looked more relaxed.

Bill had gone to the other side of the temporary wall to swing his mother onto her bedside potty. I called him to come. I felt he should be there. Hannah and I were still at Grandpa's bedside when we glanced over at Bill as he came into the doorway. As he was coming, Bill looked towards his father.

From the doorway where he had stopped he said, "I saw his spirit leave. He just died."

Hannah and I looked at Grandpa. He had expired. He had slipped out without the dreaded obstruction. He had scored a final victory over "Moeller Luck." He was home free.

We offered another *Our Father* for yet another departed family elder. Babe had died only two months earlier, and I hoped she was at the end of his tunnel to greet him on the other side. I imagined them laughing together again and exchanging their old stories.

As Grandpa's worn-out body awaited the hearse, I wondered what to do about Grandma. Her husband had just died, and she no longer knew she had one. Though it made little sense, I needed to take her to say good-bye to him. Perhaps it would register for her on some important level.

I guided her to stand beside his bed. She looked down at him.

"I don't like this," she announced, and turned to leave.

I helped her back to her room. I felt very strange. I had no answers, but lots of questions.

Grandma was soon fast asleep in her recliner. She had no questions. I closed her door slightly so she would not be roused by the commotion of Grandpa's bodily departure. This also filled my own need, a need to protect her feelings in case she had any.

I always presumed she could hear when we talked in front of her. I spoke as if her feelings might be hurt by something we said. There was no way of knowing definitively whether or not she might connect to herself for a moment and understand or become distraught. I guess, whether it mattered to her or not, it was good for the progression of my sensitivity to maintain respect for her once conscious humanity.

She did not attend the service at the funeral home with our family and her daughter Jane. Her oldest daughter, Rachel, who had never yet in her life attended a wake, was sick with flu and could not come.

Grandma attended the little party we held at our home right after the funeral, but she didn't know it.

Beyond Endurance

Grandma rested in her recliner, an ever-present tissue locked into her coiled fingers. Supposedly it was for her drippy nose, but she liked to shred it. When it was in bits on the floor, she'd point to the box of Kleenex and indicate her desire for another one.

She expressed her wants with pantomime as words escaped her. She was beginning to forget how to chew and then swallow. She could not be left alone to eat, and her food was prepared without lumps.

She no longer remembered to push a bit in order to accomplish a bowel movement. Hannah taught me to sit Grandma on her potty, put on rubber gloves, and apply pressure at a certain place on Grandma's bottom, which generally produced success. If anyone had told me when I was twenty that I'd be popping poop from my mother-in-law's bum someday, I might have given up on life entirely. However, it's amazing what can become just another routine.

Following Grandpa's August funeral, Grandma's relentless dementia continued its ravaging path. She remained gentle and compliant as her illness progressed. She seemed without awareness that her life had ever been different as she sat contentedly at the kitchen table doing single piece infant puzzles by the hour. We acquired a huge stack of these wooden puzzles with a small knob on each image. These had pictures of animals, boats, birds, cars, and so forth. Carefully, she would trace each piece, and feel around every opening. Her vision was not good. As Paul watched her while on one of his caretaker relief patrols, he got the idea to paint the backgrounds black to contrast them with the puzzles' tan edges. After his creative endeavor she usually placed the piece, turned it, and completed her task more easily.

Because our grandchildren were around, we had discovered by accident the enjoyment old folks can gain from toys. Grandpa had taken pride in arranging a little farm on the kitchen table; Nonie and Babe had loved playing with puppets. Our very young and very old had so many ways they could interact and connect.

One afternoon Grandma sat forward in her recliner, reached for her walker, and used it to pull herself up. She stood there holding it.

Go," she commanded the walker.

When it refused to take her anywhere, she sat back down again.

She never attempted to walk through the thing as Nonie had done, so I didn't take it away from her. She was still able to walk, and I thought it might be more dangerous for her to try without it. As persons are unique, so it seems, is the way an illness affects a particular individual.

She pointed to her bed. I guided her there, helped her lie down and elevated the side-rails. We had rented a hospital bed for the very reason that it had them to protect her from tumbling out and breaking another bone. Soon she fell fast asleep.

When I was sure Grandma was snoring soundly, I went over to check my mother. When I was without help from Hannah or the Visiting Nurses I often had to switch back and forth between the two of them.

My mother's legs continued to become weaker and more painful, even as her head drooped more and more. She really needed a wheelchair but would not accept one. She could no longer lift her left leg, and dragged it along on the inner arch of the foot. I pulled up her support stockings every morning, and Bill extracted her from them every evening. She hollered less at him, and he performed the task matter-of-factly and efficiently. By nightfall her legs had become very swollen, and pulling off that tight hosiery was a gristly task.

Both day and night my mother was in pain from the legs she continued to overuse, and her incessant cries would waft through the open windows into the warm September air.

"Mary, Mary, Heeellllllpp, Damnittohell, Maarrrrrry ..."

I would go into her apartment and get hold of whatever she may have been trying to reach, help her up out of a chair, or accomplish whatever task would give her peace for a moment. If I was caring for Grandma without help, she had to wait and howl for a few minutes.

Early one morning, a sensitive, young, home-health aide from the Visiting Nurses ran into my kitchen. Tears streamed down her face, and she was trembling. She had just been tending *The Mother*.

"Mrs. Donovan insisted on taking a shower," she wept, "and when she started to collapse in there she yelled at me to get behind her and catch her. I managed to get her clean, safe and dressed, but *I quit*. I can't help your mother. I'm sorry. I enjoyed coming here. You are nice people, but I quit."

Until this moment I had no idea my mother expected to be caught as part of her care. I expressed sorrow to the young woman for her awful experience and assured her I understood how she felt, and that we would miss her.

My mother abhorred the notion of germs on her body. She demanded a shower every day, and the aides only came three times a week. Her commands went unanswered partly because I could not manage her in the shower. Now, one by one, neither could the home-health aides. She was anything but the featherweight Nonie had been. She was a very heavy woman who would become deadweight when her legs gave out, and the handicapped shower stall with two side benches didn't help her. She could still prop herself up with her walker, but the walker did not fit into the shower. She would not sit on a shower chair as Grandpa had done because she had decided they were unsteady. So we learned that she insisted she was able to take a shower with the aides ready to catch her if she began to go down. She was the only person who believed this was possible, but apparently that had not altered her dictates. She would not entertain the possibility of sponge baths. Except for Babe, our resident elderly had come to enjoy their sponge baths eventually, but my mother did not believe they accomplished proper cleanliness.

She was wearing heavy-duty Depends for bathroom emergencies, but these were not always sufficient. She was becoming unable to get herself out of bed in time to reach the toilet, occasionally creating a wretched disaster.

Life was becoming intolerable. She could do little other than rant and rage, which she did well, demanding that we adjust the world to her liking. More and more she could do less and less until she ranted almost incessantly.

During these weeks of intense activity centered on my mother, Grandma's gentle and compliant nature let us fit in all the care she needed, with the help of the Visiting Nurses, Hannah, and the scraps of time and energy we would snatch away from the ordeal that was my mother.

The nurse in charge of her program planned a special visit to address the difficulties. When she arrived she found my mother dragging herself around while holding onto the sink and chairs, rather than using her walker as required. She discussed these safety issues and then confronted her with problems the home-health aides were having with her. She set out a list of requirements my mother would have to follow if the services were to continue.

The Mother appeared to listen, but then broke all the rules. She continued to demand a shower with a body-catcher. She was again caught dragging herself around without a walker. She still refused a wheelchair. Thus, the social worker for the visiting nurses came to inform her that they were required to remand her to a nursing home placement. My mother was furious, but she was running out of options.

Concurrent with the social worker's visit, Ellen arrived. We understood that a total care facility would have to be found, and so began an urgent and extensive nursing home research project. We visited every nursing home in the area, finding problems with most and becoming aghast at conditions in many. We created a mental notepad to consult each time we approached a facility. It contained the following points of inquiry and these questions became very important to us.

> Were they open to our unexpected visit?
> How did the place smell as we entered, and as we moved through it?
> Were the residents clean and cleaned up?
> How many residents were stuffed into one room?
> Was a registered nurse on duty at all times over the weekend?
> What was the client/staff ratio?
> What recreational activities were provided?
> Could each resident obtain cable TV?
> Might a resident install a personal phone?
> Did they cope with grievances in a family context?

The personal phone line and cable TV might not be important to many potential residents, but they would be essential for her. Two facilities held the promise of meeting our mother's needs. We convinced her to examine them with us, telling her how much more control she would have over her life if she could choose her own placement rather than have the nurses place her somewhere.

We used the family wheelchair and struggled to get her in and out of the car. It was nearly impossible, and after it all she was totally dissatisfied with both. She wanted her placement connected to a hospital.

Ellen departed for Connecticut to address family responsibilities, but promised to return quickly.

Screams from the apartment became ever more piercing and persistent. Somehow my mother's *Myasthenia gravis* and her arthritis were interacting to create extreme discomfort. Her medications could not be increased without the treatment for one condition creating problems for another. The visiting nurses were accomplishing little. Hannah also attempted to help, but the sufferer could not be appeased. We cooked meals for her and did what little we could.

Ellen reappeared and was given her own bedroom. She was determined to stay until we found a nursing home. We expanded our research to encompass more territory and finally found a new facility with openings. It was across the street from an excellent hospital. This nursing home, though still in Massachusetts, would also be relatively convenient for Ellen's family to visit. We knew we would never find anything better, and we were determined to get her in.

So on a bright, cheerful Sunday afternoon, while our mother was crying out in pain and unable to walk, we told her we were taking her for emergency pain evaluation. With the wheelchair and Bill's help we placed her in my car. We transported her to the emergency room of the hospital across from the targeted nursing home. Somehow we got her out of the car, into the wheelchair and into the ER. She bitched vociferously as the hospital personnel attempted to move her onto the table. When they touched her she reacted with loud yowls. The staff seemed to become completely frustrated with their inability to manage her and told us to bring her back to a specialist on Monday.

That never happened because I lost it! I broke down completely and cried the most overwhelmed, frightened and exhausted tears of my lifetime. I told them I did not even know how we'd get her back into my car, let alone how I could possibly care for her any longer. If this had been a theatrical performance, I'm sure I would not have evoked any sympathy. Hospitals see too much tragedy all the time. But this was not any sort of manipulative melodrama. I was honestly a completely wiped-out human being.

On some level I knew that children are not legally responsible for their parents. By law, I could have walked out of the hospital and told the staff I'd done the best I could and wished them luck, but I couldn't do that. I had inherited responsibility for her from my father, and his spirit had remained with me through these years of service. He had believed she was "basically good," and to honor his memory I needed to respect the goodness he had perceived, even when I couldn't feel it myself. Despite his shortcomings, he remained my primary role model for a holy and loyal life.

Ellen and I confessed to the ER staff how desperately we had hoped they'd keep her for pain evaluation, establish what would help her most, and then place her in the new nursing home across the street.

They empathized and wanted to help, but informed us our wish could not be realized without a doctor to take her as a permanent patient. On a weekend, they informed us, no doctor would be found to accept new patients.

However, after considerable calling around, they did coax a doctor to the ER. He actually agreed to assume responsibility for our mother. He was a very religious man who had dedicated much of his life to foreign missions, and perhaps we afforded him yet another spiritual opportunity. Whatever tensions we came to have with him in the future, in hindsight they are all forgiven in our gratitude for this moment!

After an in-patient evaluation, our mother was settled in the nursing home of our choice under the care of her new doctor. We informed her previous doctor, who had treated all our elders, and was still Bill's mother's doctor. She was both understanding and relieved. She had not had an easy time with *The Mother*.

I remembered sitting in her waiting room while she examined my mother. Although I accompanied the other old folks in to see her, my mother never wanted me to hear any medical evaluation. Suddenly her doctor burst into the waiting room and sat down next to me.

"I gave up and left her sitting on the examining table talking to me endlessly," admitted the poor woman, who had then given me her evaluation.

Now, cheerfully, she promised to send all records immediately.

Bill and I installed a television and phone in my mother's new room, marked and brought her clothes, and packed up many of her favorite books to arrange into a small bookcase.

She had lived in her apartment for over four years, but now never mentioned missing it. She never asked about the birds or flowers she had so enjoyed outside her sliding glass door. Surviving the distress of her diseases and adjusting to her necessary placement consumed her energy. She seemed more comfortable.

She had to adapt to a wheelchair, which removed enough stress from her legs that she was no longer in constant pain. The nursing home staff wheeled her effortlessly under an open shower. They pushed her to the dining hall. She had the total care she needed, seemed less frightened now that it was all established, and settled into the structured routine.

Ellen and I set up a visitation schedule, and she had company at least once a week. We hauled her to local restaurants to dine with her grandchildren. Each week we attempted to fill her list of desired foods and other special items. Although her demands seemed endless, I was able to go home and sleep without her screams piercing the night.

Despite having settled into a routine, *The Mother* remained unable to get along with others. Ellen or I, or both of us, received requests to meet with the nursing staff each time we'd visit. We were told that if they had not come to respect us, and appreciate our help, they would not have been able to keep her. They did not even make money from her care because she qualified for Medicaid. They were aware she was unusually difficult, though we never disclosed anything about her history. Her belligerent manner towards the aides and nursing staff made them seek to avoid her. She considered herself superior to the other residents, and treated most with arrogant antagonism.

Finding her a lasting roommate was impossible, and she went through many. Finally they experimented with a retired teacher who was able to defend her space. In silence they came to value each other to some degree. Well, sometimes it was not silent. I recall a visit when *The Mother* was blasting the Metropolitan Opera over her TV. Her roommate had a baseball game booming. They fought on, testing who was going to drown out whom.

I left them to their turf war to avoid becoming deaf and instead went to console the head nurse regarding her episode list of the week. I suggested she might become less frustrated with my mother if she thought of her as a four-year-old child and not as an adult.

"What kind of a mother was she to you and Ellen growing up?" she asked.

"Emotionally we never experienced mothering from her," I answered. "Fortunately for us we knew other nurturing persons."

"Amazing," she said, "when I consider how many sweet old mothers roam around here without a single visitor."

Speak Only to Grandma

Bill came home carrying a securely taped, foot-square brown cardboard box. It contained Grandpa's ashes, and he carried it into Grandma's room. We had decided his dust would remain with her for the time being.

No one had ever arrived in this condition. I didn't have any experience with human ashes, although I'd grown up hearing the story of Harvey.

Harvey had been my dad's banking client. As executor for Harvey's trust, my father inherited the job of sprinkling his ashes over the Atlantic from an airplane. My father had never journeyed into the clouds. In preparation for the ascent and decent, my father, a friend, and Harvey stopped by a favorite pub. They each ordered a scotch, and then each ordered a scotch for Harvey, who had been placed between them. After awhile they left for the airport. But they forgot Harvey and left him at the bar. The story always ended there. I never did hear what happened to him.

I knew what happened to Grandpa. His remains now rested on top of Grandma's bureau. I went over and stared. So much strength, so much absolutism, and so much warmth reduced to this size! Oh, I knew his spirit was not trapped within this cardboard box, but Ash Wednesday would never be the same for me. I gained some courage and lifted the carton and was shocked. It was very heavy.

I went to the kitchen and began to prepare dinner.

A few moments later I heard Grandma coming towards me. Thump, shuffle-shuffle marched the walker followed by her feet. She pivoted herself around the walker with one hand, and looked into my face.

"Who may I ask are you?"

"I'm Mary who married your son, Bill. I'm Mary of 'Mary and Bill.' You live in our house, and we are taking care of you."

"And who, may I ask, am I?" asked Grandma.

"You are Cecilia Leuper. You married Will Moeller, and became Cecilia Moeller."

"I am Cecilia Leuper."

Satisfied, she thumped and shuffled her way back to her room and melted into her recliner. She pulled her favorite blanket over her and was soon fast asleep.

Perhaps a week later, Bill left for an evening meeting at our town hall, and I was alone with Grandma. She was sleeping in her hospital bed with the side-rails elevated, and I was in the kitchen reading the newspaper. When the home-health aide had come a short while earlier, she had not been able to rouse Grandma from a deep sleep, so I'd let her leave early.

Suddenly I heard the bed-rail rattling. As I entered her room, I saw Grandma throwing her leg over the metal bar, attempting to swing herself as if it were gymnastics equipment. I put the rail down and pivoted her to her potty. She piddled. I escorted her to her recliner and brought some food and drink. She was not interested and told me that there was a man in a red suit in her room. She motioned as if he were to her right, and then tried to get up out of the chair. I guided her back to bed, put the rail up, and left to continue reading believing she would doze off again as usual. Vigorously, she began to shake the bar again and by the time I returned to the room she had nearly swung herself over the edge and onto the floor.

I put the side down and sat on the edge of the bed with my back towards her. With tremendous strength Grandma pushed against me, trying to force her way through me. Then she started speaking in a deep, deep voice.

"I always did my best. I supported my family."

This did not sound like Grandma. It was not her voice. Roughly she grabbed my hand in a vise grip and pushed it into her crotch.

"Look what I have for you," the deep voice declared.

"Grandma," I said, "why don't you lie back and rest."

"I am a good man," came the low-toned utterance.

Grandma continued to thrash against my back, almost pushing me off the bed.

I began to feel helpless, frightened and a bit spooked. I was not going to respond to the guttural speech. That tone didn't sound like any Grandma I'd ever known.

"Would you like something to drink, Grandma?" I asked.

"You wouldn't give me what I want to drink," answered the voice.

I thought I would lose the battle, and Grandma would throw herself on the floor and break another bone. Hysteria turned my stomach, and I remembered how I'd felt this way while caring for Nonie.

"Relax, breathe, and give birth to your peace. Relax, breathe, and give birth to transcendence. Relax, breathe, and give birth to your Love," I urged myself once again.

I remembered the Holy Family pictured on the wall of my bedroom when I was young. I had not thought about that image for years. The Child played in the light of love and the monsters could not touch Him. He had not seemed to notice them, and certainly had not given them the least attention.

Grandma continued thrashing forcefully against my back, but I felt calmer and more in command.

"I worked hard. I did the best I could," intoned the voice.

"Grandma, aren't you tired?" I asked.

We continued this barter until Bill returned from the town hall and found me sitting on the edge of his mother's bed. After greeting me, and hearing I'd had a hard time, he asked his mother if she would like a drink.

"Yes, yes," she said ever so sweetly.

I left Grandma with Bill, and retired.

A few days later the hospice volunteer arrived for my reprieve. She came once a week. She went into Grandma's room, passed her as she slept in bed, and seated herself in the recliner. Comfortable, she turned to me and confided that Grandpa's spirit was present in the room. I bristled, knowing I had not mentioned my experience to her or to any of the nursing staff.

"What do you mean?" I asked.

"Oh I can tell when he's here. Sometimes he even gets into Grandma. You see, Alzheimer's patients have so little mind left when they are dying that they become excellent mediums for spirits," she explained.

"Are you, Grandma, and Grandpa going to be okay for a while together? Would you rather not hang out with spirits?" I asked.

"Oh, heavens, I'm used to it. I'll be just fine. Go along and get some rest," she instructed.

As I left the room I glanced over at Grandpa's ashes.

"Chill out," I silently commanded. "She'll be with you soon enough."

Family Connections

We were an extended family of the living and the dead. Welcoming the ancient relatives had joined our families in a common dance. I realized that friends, family members, and even the deceased were contained within me and enhanced my personal uniqueness.

While Nonie was dying, and constantly calling, "Mary," occasionally she would evoke, "Mum." She and Babe had remarked how much I'd remind them of their mother. Although I never met my grandmother, I'd been told all my life that when my dad first saw my newborn form he'd said, "She looks just like Mum."

As Mum or I were alternately summoned to Nonie's bedside, I felt this ancestor present to her dying children through my apparent resemblance to her. Sometimes it was a pleasant feeling, as when Nonie would seem soothed by her mother's attention.

The process of caring for our dying elders had brought my sister and me closer together. The continuing responsibility for our mother had settled us into the same vessel.

We had never been a close-knit sister duo, as we were rarely in the same place at the same time during childhood. We had very different experiences of our parents and dissimilar defense mechanisms for coping with our difficult family circumstances. Consequently, if Ellen and I, with our history of interpersonal distance, could benefit from working together for our elders, I had hoped Bill and his sisters might also experience a deeper relationship. As Grandma's Alzheimer's progressed, I dreamt they might find some comparable bond through common service.

It's always risky to dream about what might benefit others without discussing these goals with them. Whenever I've usurped another's potential as my concern it has become apparent that my vision of their potential is not what they had in mind. I know that we are each responsible for ourselves, and that the most I can do for another is trek beside them at their pace. As a therapist I must be careful not to impose my concept of another's realization but to remain but a catalyst for their perspective about personal growth. Each person's maturation has its own beats and pauses. So although I should have known better, my dream for a deeper relationship between Bill and his sisters not only imaged my vision but also specified its realization on my time schedule.

The relationship between Bill and his sisters did not improve as we cared for his mother. They did not live nearby, and Jane visited less often now that her father had died. Rachael kept in touch by phone. Both wrote disturbing letters critiquing our care. They seemed to believe that their mother's problems were caused by our inadequate attention, and how much money we spent on the effort was constantly questioned. It was exhausting at a time when we got little sleep.

I wondered if the family dynamics might improve if I stepped out of the middle and had Bill communicate directly with his sisters. Because I was the primary caregiver, I felt I might stand between Bill and a better relationship with them. After I discussed this with him he wrote the following letter to both Jane and Rachel:

> With regard to a need for any discussion on matters dealing with our mother, I request that all communications be directly between us, her children, and that all others remain

outside the loop. The recent experiences in this house condition me to this request. When Mary's Mother, Babe, and Nonie were here in our care and under similar circumstances to Mom's, we all worked from a never-explicitly-stated understanding that I was non-family and thus had no role other than to be a physical presence and muscular strength to be used to assist at whatever times and in whatever ways Mary and Ellen deemed appropriate at any stage of their caring for them. The sisters were able, without having to factor me into the dynamic, to work out their division of labor in providing physical and emotional care and were also free to deal with those unsettled matters of the life-histories within their family that the approach of those deaths brought up between any of the five of them. We all lived through the progress of those deaths; or in the case of Mary's Mother, her placement and ongoing residence in an intensive-care nursing home situation, very comfortably. It worked (is working) very well. On all sides, respect and understanding flourished, and thus the dying were physically and emotionally supported in a peaceful environment.

Although some tensions are obvious between us as we live beyond Dad's death and through our mother's dying, please be assured and feel comfortable that you are welcome here whenever you might wish to come.

If more seems worth the risk, great, for I, too, share the hope that has been often enough stated in the last year or so: that we might come to greater understanding, respect, and appreciation of ourselves and each other as we live our way through the penultimate death on our family trees."

Rachel wrote back to Bill:

I agree wholeheartedly with your suggestion that we three discuss matters dealing with our mother. Perhaps this will be the beginning of something good.

It was not.

I felt really sad. At this point I reckoned the harmony I had wanted for this family was not going to happen, and hoped my own exhaustion with the situation had not made things worse. How I had desired peace and community!

Perhaps there is nothing as divisive as the grieving process when members of the same family, suffering the same loss, find themselves isolated in different corners unable to comfort each other. One may deny anything is wrong while another is angry about the suffering. One may need quiet surroundings while another may feel better lost in bursts of noisy activity. One may become numb and traumatized while another more reality-centered than ever before. They can do little for each other but embrace their different needs and diverse reactions. With time, acceptance may come and then family members might become closer for having survived together.

My desire for immediate harmony served my own self-interest. Life would have been more pleasant if everyone joined the same choir. I would have had only Grandma to tend and not her children's conflicts also.

On an afternoon when Rachel called, Grandma ordered the walker to take her to the phone, perhaps in response to the ring. Rachel had hoped to talk with her mother, but her mother did not wish to converse with her. Grandma's thoughts were elsewhere.

"I have a load in my pants," she announced.

"I heard that," Rachel said before resuming her conversation.

She may have heard it intellectually, but she did not smell it. I didn't believe she had any concept of what it was going to take to clean Grandma.

Because money seemed so important to the sisters I considered submitting a bill for my services but dismissed the notion as stemming from my annoyance. But it may not have been a bad idea, as it might have helped me feel less subservient to the problems of this conflicted crew!

Poor vulnerable Grandma was my big baby now. Sometimes she slept curled into a fetal position resembling a boney, wizened infant.

Caring for her did not dredge up old baggage, as did caring for my relatives. She was not a part of my childhood and did not place me face to face with the forces that influenced my development or lack thereof. Oh, I had blamed her over the years for some of Bill's quirks. Mothers can be unfairly blamed for their children's habits. But this was not as intense as colliding with my own past, from which I did not yet have enough distance to allow me compassion for Bill's sisters' struggles. While moving to accept their father's death and all he had been or had not been to their lives, they now had to face the death of their mother soon thereafter.

Matters only became more embroiled when the distant sisters began to believe we were threatening their mother's welfare by not feeding her on a regular schedule. Grandma had deteriorated to the point where she slept a great deal of the time, and was rarely hungry. Her body was beginning the natural process of shutting down in preparation for death, as disease was destroying her brain. Those who do not understand the dying process fear this is painful and want to insert a feeding tube to prevent hunger. I'm sure such medical interventions create more pain and confusion as they disrupt a natural blunting process in preparation for the final farewell. Fortunately Grandma had explicitly written out what she wanted, or didn't want, during her competent days on earth.

My sleeping fetus would suddenly uncurl and resurrect from deep unconsciousness with an appetite at strange times, such as ten in the evening or two in the morning. Then she might want a liverwurst sandwich accompanied by ginger ale, and we would prepare this meal for her. It was safer to give her food when she was alert enough to eat because this diminished her tendency to choke. But the sisters insisted nothing was wrong with her, and that she was just undergoing some elderly decline, some "senile dementia" that comes with old age. They were not able to hear anything about an illness and its sequence. Therefore, Grandma's mental and physical degeneration became more and more our fault.

Grandma's conscientious medical doctor, who had already become familiar with the family as she'd ministered to Grandpa, wanted to gather them together to discuss her patient's disease and it's progression. She petitioned Bill, Jane, Rachel and me to assemble for a conference in her office. She hoped to have the sisters dialogue with her, learn, and have their concerns addressed in a family context, where the stress Bill and I lived with would also be acknowledged.

This meeting never came to pass. Rachel and Jane had only visited together for Grandpa's last birthday, and arranging travel for such an engagement was not a priority.

One afternoon, a few months before Grandma died, Jane arrived and sat in a chair beside her mother's recliner. She spoke in a deep tone requesting rich confidences.

"Mother, tell me the truth. Brother Bill was an accident wasn't he?"

I was working in the kitchen a short distance away and could not help but overhear her question. I admit I stepped slightly to one side so I could watch my mother-in-law's reaction.

She remained, as she had been, blank-faced and unresponsive, locked in demented silence.

How I wished she could speak. I knew from years of discourse with her that this mother had rejoiced in welcoming her son.

Very Young and Very Old

Bill and I never sheltered our children from the actuality of death. We knew that in many societies children play alongside all aspects of life, and death's realization coats perspective. We believed our own society attempts to shadow that reality by segregating the terminally ill, through an idolization of youthful sexuality, by investing in technologies of immortality, and the continuous production of cosmetic innovations to disguise the aging process.

When Peter, our oldest child was only a bit over two, he accompanied us to his granduncle's wake. The family was surprised when we lifted such a young child to look into the casket and view the face of death. Peter's bright eyes glistened as he gazed upon the deceased, vacuuming the cosmic encounter into his young consciousness. We have always adhered to the position that interaction with reality was beneficial and often healing.

My grandsons arrived three days a week throughout the years I tended the dying. Nurturing their young lives towards a future beyond my own time balanced my farewells to the past.

As they were able, the boys and I listened to children's music, often accompanying it with a rhythm band. We played ball outside in the sun, read many books and told stories. We played by the hour with a large castle; lining up brave knights, hiding princesses from dragons, and saving children lost in forests endangered by imagined wild animals, ghosts or spooky trees. Yet, they understood when I had to take a break to change an adult diaper or prepare a snack for the ancient ones.

Trevor had been two when his brother Erik came into our world one week after Nonie had died. He was over three years old when Babe died.

He had loved both Babe and Nonie, and they had chuckled heartily while playing with him. However, as Babe began to fail, he seemed to sense another death coming and began to avoid her.

Upon her death, he became nasty towards me. He snapped his precise little sentences in my direction and would not hug me anymore. He dismissed me.

I felt hurt and confused. We'd been such good friends. Then one day I was startled by my reflection in the mirror. I observed my gray hair, and the fact that I looked a bit like Babe. I guessed the problem between my elder grandson and me.

When visiting his home one evening I said to him, "You think I'm going to die like Babe died don't you? I bet that is why you've been so mean to me."

"That's right," he said.

"Well, I can't promise you I won't die," I said. "Mama can't promise me she won't die. But if she died I'd cry and cry and cry, but then I would go on living, because life is beautiful while we have it. It is our treasure."

"So if you died or Mama died I'd go on living," exclaimed Trevor.

"You would be sad, but you would survive," I said.

"So if Mama dies, you would live and if you die Mama will live, and if you die I will live, and if I die Mama will live, and if Mama dies I will live, and this is the truth of the law," proclaimed Trevor

"Sounds good," said I, wondering if his paternal grandfather's law degree was genetic.

We hugged and became friends again.

When Grandpa began his severe decline immediately after Babe died, I kept the little ones upstairs or outside, and away from him as much as possible.

While Erik was napping one afternoon, I told Trevor I'd begin to teach him to play chess. He seemed excited about this. Our employee, Helen, heard us and expressed her interest in learning the epic game. She asked Trevor to teach her after he knew how to play.

Trevor and I climbed upstairs to the family room and sat on the floor. I placed my father's old chessboard between us, and I began to instruct him as I had been taught, and as I had taught my children before him.

He had been concentrating very hard for quite some time when he suddenly jumped up.

"Just a minute, Nanny," he said, and took off.

He went to the head of the stairs and called down to Helen, who quickly stood below him.

"Helen," he shouted definitively, "I won't be able to teach you how to play chess today."

Upon Grandpa's death I encountered yet another dilemma with Trevor.

When Grandpa had first come to our home he'd been very affectionate to Trevor, but later came to dismiss this dark-eyed, dark-haired boy. He was "not a Moeller" like his little blond, blue-eyed brother, for whom Grandpa made his preference very obvious. His general disposition, now compounded by terminal illness, could dismiss another easily.

Trevor had been hurt by his great-grandfather's rejection, and said he was glad he'd died. We assured him it was fine and good to honor his feelings and admit to us that he would be relieved by Grandpa's absence. Honest ownership of negative feelings helps move us all beyond our hurts to embrace the best of another. Eventually Trevor was able to remember fun times with Grandpa and understand that cancer poisons had influenced his hurtful behavior.

As an adult I had often felt overwhelmed by the stressful behavior of the dying person and found it hard to remember the essence of my loved one. When Nonie died I had felt relieved for her and for myself that the high-pitched screaming had ended. Often the best of Nonie seemed long forgotten as we struggled with the paranoia of her dementia. Yet I soon had learned, as Trevor learned, that the spirit of a lost one springs back once the suffering is over. The more time passes and the deeper the personal bond to the deceased, the clearer the memory of all the pleasant times becomes.

The children ripened for an entire year before another death loomed before us. It was then old Grandma's turn to fade dramatically.

Grandma was the only ancient person little Erik remembers, but more as a distant image because he did not feel close to her. She was beyond any capacity for relationship when this bright, cheerful two-year-old formed conscious memories.

As she slept more and more, the home-health aides could do little for Grandma during their time with us, and so Erik enjoyed slipping into her room and enticing them to play with him instead of twiddling their time away with an immoveable patient. He often succeeded in diverting them, and developed a special fondness for a few younger workers. He had a fantastic ability to inspire laughter. His incredible language skills enabled him to define the world around him in a refreshing fashion, which delighted everyone.

I was not concerned about Erik and the loss of his great-grandmother. I knew he would miss a few of those young aides more than he would miss her, but Trevor was set up for yet another death.

Therefore, on a sunny day in August when Grandma had an appointment with our medical doctor, Bill and I packed Trevor into our car along with her. After the exam, we discussed Grandma with the doctor in his presence. I explained all the family deaths he remembered, and how he had lost some special friends. Our discerning doctor sat Trevor on her lap and told him how privileged he was to have had an opportunity to experience life in context. She reminded him of his brother's birth, and offered her hope that he would be able to envision the whole scope of life, from birth to death. She indicated that peering through such a wide lens could expand his awareness of the beauty and meaning of existence.

Trevor listened with his usual intense concentration, and appeared profoundly impressed. He was never as close to any of the elders as he had been to Babe, so it may have been easier for him to fathom the doctor's words in the company of Bill's mother. She sat through all of this in her wheelchair, focusing upon nothing at all, comprehending nothing at all.

We arrived back home and unpacked the car. Bill wheeled Grandma to her room and turned her over to Hannah, who had been with Erik as he napped. Trevor and I went to our upstairs haven and played with the castle. He buried some gray-headed figures under grass and rocks and found a group of kids to jump on them. Then the knights came and carried the children off to play with their parents inside the castle walls. When Erik woke up he found the buried ones and brought them back to life. Trevor begrudgingly allowed this!

Imaginative play is a well-known outlet for children's feelings, and it was fun to watch this in action.

We switched to a musical activity and played a few lively CDs. The children and I created a hullabaloo with the rhythm instruments and enjoyed our fun.

The very young had given the very old a great many laughs. The very old had given the very young a sense of their history, and exposure to the seasons of life. Those of us lodged somewhere in the middle were able to look in both directions and smile.

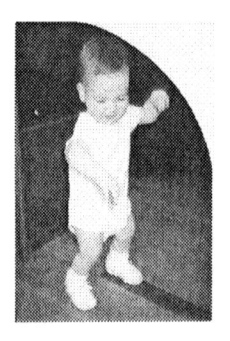

Trevor Dancing

Free Spirit

Old Grandma was becoming like an ever-sleeping infant who had not yet learned to smile. Seized in Alzheimer's grip, her brain was gradually shutting down. She was not in pain. Generally, she was not agitated. She entered a near-comatose state, and when she occasionally did become agitated, she would rise up in her bed as a voiceless, expressionless, rigid form summoning surreal images of the resurrection of the dead.

At such times we would focus on assuring her comfort. Was she hungry? Was she thirsty? Did she need her potty? Was she cold? She could not tell us.

She never required a single invasive tube. Bill lifted her onto her potty several times a day. It amazed me that this ritual worked even when she seemed to be in an unconscious state. A home-health aide and I were standing at the foot of her bed when he raised her yet one more time. From where we stood it looked as if he was lifting a corpse right out of a coffin. We asked him not to do it anymore. We both felt that she should no longer be disturbed. We said we'd simply change her when necessary.

Grandma was comatose.

Hannah or I kept her mouth moist with little wet sponge lollipops and her lips oiled so they would not dry out and crack. She seemed comfortable and at peace.

The very evening following our decision to let her be, she began the now familiar irregular breathing pattern. I gathered some pillows and blankets and settled myself into her recliner for the night. I didn't want her to die alone, even if she seemed oblivious to my presence. Sometimes I talked to her and prayed out loud, in case she could hear me. If she could hear me, then maybe she would know she was not alone. At a basic level we all die alone, as we are born alone, gasping our own last breath as our first, but by being there I was aware of my attempt to honor her unique life. Though there is so much we must experience alone we are, nonetheless, social beings.

Bill slept upstairs, as he had a class to teach in the morning. We determined her status had not changed by morning, so he went off to give his lecture. In our experience, the dying had hung on with this weird breathing for days. Grandma did not. She died a few hours later. One breath was simply the last.

I called Bill, but she had been pronounced and her body removed by the time he was able to get home. He had already said good-bye to her, so this did not bother him. The release of her body was an afterdeath. Whatever thread that had held her spirit captive to this world was now severed, and she was free.

When our loved ones died a little bit each day, and more and more each month, we found we grieved a little bit each day, and a little more each month. The sorrow spreads out over time instead of being encapsulated in an intense experience of loss. By the time Grandma died, only the silent molecules of her shape remained to be taken from us.

When Bill arrived home he gathered tools from his shop by the garage and with conscious symbolic effort, took down the temporary wall he had constructed when Babe and Nonie were headed our way three years earlier. He did this almost as he walked into the house, representing the end of our service to the dying.

The hospital bed was returned to its rental company and we threw out the recycled recliner. We readied the house for a party to celebrate Bill's parents' lives and our gratitude to all the nurses and home-health aides who had supported us over the past years.

The party began with a wake and religious service for Bill's mom at the funeral home. Jane and Rachel arrived with their spouses. Rachel, though well into her sixties, crept into the funeral parlor looking like an unsure child.

"What do I do?" she asked me. "I've never been to one of these before."

Jane had attended her father's funeral but Rachel had been too ill. As she and I knelt together before the open casket, I felt a deep sadness. What must it be like to face the dead for the first time in your sixties and in relation to your own mother? I looked over at my grandsons playing underneath the chairs and felt grateful they might be able to see their lives in context from beginning to earthly completion. Yes, we are all but "dust, and unto dust we will return." We are destined to lose many a loved one's embrace as well as every material thing.

I seated myself among the chairs before Grandma's coffin, and reflected upon my own life. Had I freed myself from the idolization of transient delights, while still relishing all the earthy beauty my consciousness could hold? With profound gratitude I thought about loved ones with whom I had grown up over many years. They were my life's joy, and my love for them would be the only armor I would carry when it came my time to journey beyond death.

Father Bob and Sister Roberta led the group in song and prayer as we assembled together, until it was time to offer a last farewell and return to our home.

In recognition of Grandma and Grandpa, everyone had a great time. We expressed our thanks to many. Bill's sisters expressed appreciation to Hannah for all she had done to make their parents' final days comfortable.

The siblings were civil to each other in respect for their hard-working, well-intentioned parents. The tensions of previous times were put aside in this desire to honor the dead and the history of a family.

Eventually Bill brought home yet another heavy, brown, square box. A short while later he placed the remains of his parents together in our cemetery plot. As youngsters from New York City I'm sure this couple never imagined they would be buried together in a small town's burying ground located in a northern state.

A Single Tear

After the celebration for Bill's parents everyone returned home. For the first time in years, there was no one else living anywhere in our home. Immediately, we adapted to our new reality! When Bill went off to the University, I was able to play my new piano without fear of waking the almost-dead. My grandsons and I romped around the whole house. Bill and I no longer needed a restaurant for a private conversation.

I called Jane to inform her that I had obtained copies of her mother's death certificate from our town hall and that I would mail them to her directly. She needed them in order to settle her parent's estate.

"What did the doctor say was the cause of death?" she asked.

"Alzheimer's disease," I answered.

"Oh," said Jane.

It was September 1996, and Bill and I gratefully enjoyed uninterrupted sleep. We enjoyed uninterrupted sleep until the telephone rang late one night, about two weeks after Grandma's death.

My mother's nursing home had called. She'd had a stroke and been taken to the Emergency Room. I had visited her a few days earlier with the items on her request list. At that time she was weak, difficult to maneuver, rather pale, and demonstrated difficulty breathing. Certainly her illness was progressing, but I had not expected a stroke. I suppose no one ever expects a stroke!

She was pathetic in the intensive care unit. Her left arm drooped, as did her whole left side to some degree, indicating damage to the right side of her brain. As a right-handed person, language ability would commonly be located in the left side of her brain. This would explain why she could still talk, and even scream as usual.

She was terrified and pitiable beyond words. A nurse could not touch her without evoking a deluge of frightened howls. When a number of hospital staff came to move her from bed to chair to stimulate her circulation, her howling could be heard far down the hospital corridor. Her every movement was a nightmare for all.

Eventually, she was returned to her nursing home's rehabilitation floor. They worked hard to recover as much of her functioning as they could, but she was not anyone's favorite patient. Her left arm did improve, and although she never completely regained the use of her hand, she could use it to steady paper or her dinner tray.

The rehab unit could only keep her so long until they had to return her to the original floor. She had been a difficult patient before the stroke. Now she was impossible. Suddenly it seemed as if my sister and I lived at the nursing home, trying to mediate as many tensions as possible, and attempting to maximize whatever good spirits we could conjure up. Though a Medicaid patient, the staff gave up trying to manage her in relationship to a roommate and placed her in private quarters.

On a visit about six weeks after the stroke, I brought my mother a big box of little, seedless Spanish oranges. She loved to share these with staff she liked and refuse them to staff she found aggravating. During this visit she insisted I take her out to a local mall so she could shop. I told her I could barely hoist her off the toilet in her large, private bathroom, and wondered how she thought I'd care for her at a mall. Her breathing was terrible, she was a dead weight, and her color was ghastly.

Before I left for the night, I asked the nurse on duty to check her because I thought she might be ill. She promised she would.

My phone rang late that night.

Yet again, my mother was in the Emergency Room.

She had fallen out of bed and broken her hip.

I stood chilled and shaking in our dark bedroom with the phone frozen into my hand. I was overwhelmed with feelings of dread and exhaustion. We had just survived the horror of her stroke. Now it was back to the hospital for what seemed liked a cruel joke.

Why weren't the side-rails on her bed raised? I requested an answer to this question.

Apparently the law stated that if a patient did not want rails raised they could not be elevated without a doctor's order. To do so would be considered unlawful restraint against a patient's wishes. Therefore, this large, barely mobile woman had slept in a twin bed, as a rock climber might be perched on the side of a mountain. She crashed, and they heard her scream.

She continued screaming until she was medicated.

The orthopedic surgeon arrived and my mother told him to do what he could for her. From that point on it didn't matter what Ellen and I said, or that I was her health care proxy. She had made her statement to the doctor.

As the surgery to repair her hip was about to begin the anesthesiologist wanted to know if I realized she had pneumonia. I had not been given this information until that moment. Could I, should I, try to stop everything at this point and tell them to keep her comfortable with morphine? Would they have listened if I had tried?

I wish I had! Instead, the young surgeon bragged about how he'd never lost a patient. But our mother almost died a number of times following the operation. When Ellen and I visited her in the ICU, she'd had every possible tube inserted. We were told stories about how they'd had to bring her back from the dead. She'd had a DNR, but somehow, it was no longer in her file. No one had seen any "Do

Not Resuscitate." It had vanished.

In a somewhat conscious moment she saw me. The corners of her mouth turned way down as she non-verbally communicated how awful it all was, how very terrifying. Once again I pictured the wretched, small child she had seemed to me as she stood beside my father's open grave.

An Intensive Care Unit nurse, who had been kind and helpful to her during the stroke merely a few weeks earlier, came towards me.

"Can you believe this?" I asked.

"No," she answered.

They moved her out of the ICU and up to the third floor of the hospital. The orthopedic surgeon kept telling my sister and me how well she was doing.

"How are her lungs?" I asked.

"Oh, they're worse. They are more filled with fluid, but often they get worse before they get better."

My sister and I looked at each other. Did the guy think we were idiots? We presumed he didn't want her to die on his statistics. He had not accurately evaluated how sick she was before he'd operated. She would have to suffer.

She screamed and screamed, though not fully conscious. We begged him to give her more medication. He would not.

"She's not suffering. I have patients up and walking around a day after surgery," he explained.

"She thinks she's suffering," I answered.

He would not budge.

My mother's howl's resounded down the hospital corridor.

"How are her blood gases?" asked Ellen.

"They're fine. She's well oxygenated, and doing better than I thought she would."

"That's because she's screaming so much," stated Ellen.

"See, good screamer's live longer," answered the doctor.

"Her pain should be treated," said Ellen.

"Then she'd stop screaming and could die. Her blood gases would not be as good," said the doctor.

"She's dying anyway," said Ellen.

Her turned and left us without comment.

This man did not represent the vocation I had so passionately wanted for myself so many years ago. Such a doctor would never have inspired me to dedicate my life to compassionate service.

Ellen and I finagled our mother out of the hospital, off his statistics, and back to the nursing home. She was given a morphine drip. She was not conscious, although she would still moan. She was dying of pneumonia, as she probably would have been anyway. Her lungs were too damaged to survive it. She was alone in a room used for medical situations.

Slowly, Ellen and I began the process of trying to get the tubes removed and a hospice perspective initiated. This was not easy, because our mother's initial doctor, who had saved us by coming to the ER two years earlier, and had remained our mother's devoted physician, did not accept the hospice mentality. He knew she was dying but believed he should do everything possible to prolong life as long as possible. The DNR was not replaced into her file. My status as health care proxy meant nothing. It seemed we discussed philosophy with this doctor endlessly. Our mother reminded him of his own mother, and he was having trouble letting her go. He told us so himself.

Finally, he removed the feeding tube. Tube by tube, Ellen and I encouraged him to leave her to God.

On a clear cold night in December, less than eight weeks after Grandma's death, Ellen and I were summoned to the nursing home. Our mother was comatose, and her vitals indicated she had little time remaining. We stood on either side of her bed and prayed the *Our Father* together. One tear appeared at the corner of our mother's eye and rolled down her cheek. Was it a real tear? Did she feel something for us or for her tragic life? Did she simply have such edema that some of the water within seeped out?

When I touched her she felt like a cold water-balloon from a children's party. Maybe all the water from the bathtub in Bellevue Hospital, where I'd left her long ago, was now contained within her.

She died.

I did not cry. Ellen cried because she felt sad that she did not want to cry.

We left the room around 3 A.M., assured that our funeral director was on his way for the fifth time. It crossed my mind that if our family ever called him again it would most likely be for Bill or me!

I turned and looked back. Florescent lights illuminated her face and made it appear bloated, shiny and inhumanly white. She looked ghastly, yet she was not complaining. I stared at her expecting her to rise up from the bed and scream. I expected a howling temper tantrum defining how she did not like this and demanding to know who had done it to her. I felt a terror, but I did not run. I waited and watched. She did not scream. She did not rise up. She did not threaten me anymore. She was not more powerful than death. She really was dead. Somehow, I felt free.

Something was sliding down my cheek. What was it? It almost tickled. I touched it and found it wet. As it slid over my lips it tasted salty. One tear after another was claimed by gravity's pull. When had I last wept? I did not know. On my pediatrician's lap so long ago? Perhaps. I'd cried when Babe died, but weeping comes from somewhere else. Wherever the source, my spirit had been numbed away from it for decades.

Time to leave her. I'd felt enough for one night. Slowly, my soul might open to itself. No rush. I was tired. Ellen and I had made it through a long ordeal, and needed to prepare for our mother's burial in the plot outside New York City. Her bones would rest alongside dust from my dad, Babe, and Nonie. Corpses are piled one above the other in that crowded field. I tried imagining how their spirits would interact in a reality beyond this world. I attempted to picture their souls intermingling and dancing into the sunset. I could not. With a deep sigh of relief, I conceded their interactions were out of my realm.

Promise Kept

So *Bluegirl*, after months of good sleep, I looked at you with fresh eyes and renewed emotion. I had always taken special care of you, but had hidden you upstairs in a corner. My excuse had been that children were afraid of you.

As I gazed upon you with rested eyes, I unexpectedly confronted my old feelings of danger and death. Now familiar tears swelled my eyes. I felt you as my mother. A shudder convulsed me as I gazed upon a picture of the violent child-woman about to destroy her own.

"I'm not afraid of you any longer," I said. "Perhaps you did your best. Perhaps we all do our best."

I took you down from the wall and almost embraced you. I looked into your eyes.

"All right, child, I love you, you poor sick little thing. I forgive you, perhaps because I survived you. Everything is fine. We can be friends."

I carried the huge painting downstairs for the first time in years, and hung it next to my precious piano. Somehow, the *Bluegirl* looked happy.

Weeks later I stood up from the piano bench grateful for a deep serenity after creating an emotive composition. As I was about to leave the room I turned back and looked at you, *Bluegirl*. Suddenly, I felt dizzy and entranced by your intense blue eyes.

"She is you," I told myself. "You were afraid of yourself."

I understood why I'd needed to marry someone I supposed could throttle me before I would ever be able to hurt him. I had harbored an inherent belief that my natural assertiveness required strong, external control lest I turn into my dangerous mother. Perhaps I had even set Bill up to become this policeman.

With immeasurable sadness I swept across a panorama of my life. I saw myself searching for the integrated and holistic feelings I'd had for Daniel, to begin with, and had buried miles underground. I felt sad for Bill, and anyone I may have hurt or confused while looking for my lost self. Yet I knew I'd loved others to the best of my ability. That's all I could do. That's all I can continue to do. Rather love with imperfection than flee from love for fear of imperfection.

I pictured my good husband, who would do anything to help anyone anytime he could. A smile crept over my soul as a hug for Daniel. I found myself trembling. Yet I stepped towards his *Bluegirl*.

"Give me that hammer child.
Come on, Bluegirl, hand it down.
I told your story. It's okay. It's okay.
I know you'll never swing that hammer.
You're free to put it aside and reach for the dangling, naked doll, that symbolic vision of your damaged self.
Weep with sorrow for all you lost. Weep with joy for all you learned. Weep with the relief of freedom and the ecstasy of feeling.
You are who you are, and your life is what it is, and all life is beautiful. You are but part of the marred human condition. Snuggle your flawed fetus into your arms.
Love and rejoice in community.
Love and serve the hardship of others.
Love and be content."